A Practical Approach to Pharmaceutical Analysis

Instrumental and Manual

for B. Pharmacy and M. Pharmacy Students

Name: ______________________

Class: ______________________ Roll No: ______________________

Subject: Pharmaceutical Analysis

Institution: ______________________

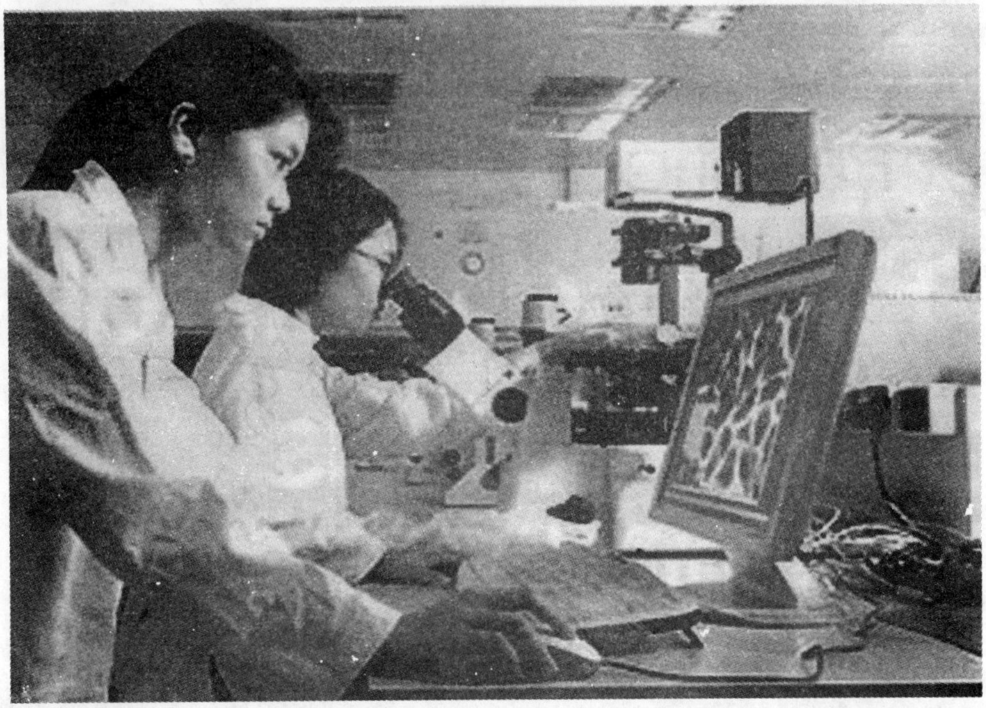

Other CBS publications by Nema *et al*

1. **Pharmaceutical Engineering Drawing** for B. Pharmacy Students
2. **Textbook of Cosmetics** for B. Pharmacy Students

A Practical Approach to Pharmaceutical Analysis

Instrumental and Manual

for B. Pharmacy and M. Pharmacy Students

Edited by

Rajesh Kumar Nema
Director, SD College of Pharmacy and Vocational Studies, Muzaffarnagar, UP

S. N. Meyyanathan
Professor and Head, Department of Pharmaceutical Analysis,
JSS College of Pharmacy, Ooty, Tamilnadu

Chandra Shekhar Sharma
Senior Lecturer, BN College of Pharmacy, Udaipur, Rajasthan

Mahesh Verma
Senior Lecturer, Faculty of Pharmacy, Integral University, Lucknow, UP

C.S. Bhan
Principal, MGCPS, Jaipur, Rajasthan

CBSPD

CBS Publishers & Distributors Pvt Ltd

New Delhi • Bengaluru • Chennai • Kochi • Kolkata • Lucknow • Mumbai
Hyderabad • Jharkhand • Nagpur • Patna • Pune • Uttarakhand

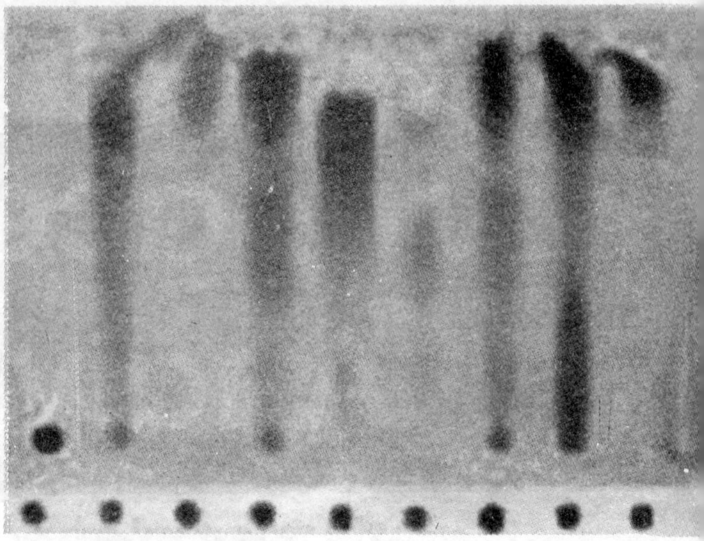

A Practical Approach to
Pharmaceutical Analysis
Instrumental and Manual
For B. Pharmacy & M. Pharmacy Students

ISBN: 978-81-239-1617-0

First Edition: 2008
Reprint: 2011, 2015, 2017, 2019, 2023 2024

Published by **Satish Kumar Jain** and produced by **Varun Jain** for
CBS Publishers & Distributors Pvt Ltd
4819/XI Prahlad Street, 24 Ansari Road, Daryaganj, New Delhi 110 002
Ph: 011-23289259, 23266861, 23266867 Fax: 011-23243014 Website: www.cbspd.com
e-mail: delhi@cbspd.com

Corporate Office: 204 FIE, Industrial Area, Patparganj, Delhi 110 092
Ph: 011-4934 4934 Fax: 011-4934 4935 e-mail: publishing@cbspd.com; publicity@cbspd.com

Branches

- **Bengaluru:** Seema House 2975, 17th Cross, KR Road, Banasankari 2nd Stage, Bengaluru 560 070, Karnataka, India
  Ph: +91-80-26771678/79 Fax: +91-80-26771680 e-mail: bangalore@cbspd.com
- **Chennai:** 7, Subbaraya Street, Shenoy Nagar, Chennai 600 030, Tamil Nadu, India
  Ph: +91-44-26680620, 26681266 Fax: +91-44-42032115 e-mail: chennai@cbspd.com
- **Kochi:** 42/1325, 1326, Power House Road, Opp KSEB, Power House, Ernakulum Kochi 682 018, Kerala, India
  Ph: +91-484-4059061-65,67 Fax: +91-484-4059065 e-mail: kochi@cbspd.com
- **Kolkata:** 147, Hind Ceramics Compound, 1st Floor, Nilgunj Road, Belghoria, Kolkata-700056, West Bengal, India
  Ph: +91-9096713055/7798394118, 9836841399 e-mail: kolkata@cbspd.com
- **Lucknow:** Basement, Khushnuma Complex, 7 Meerabai Marg (Behind Jawahar Bhawan),Lucknow-226001, UP, India
  Ph: +0522-4000032 e-mail: tiwari.lucknow@cbspd.com
- **Mumbai:** PWD Shed, Gala no 25/26, Ramchandra Bhatt Marg, Next to JJ Hospital Gate no. 2, Opp. Union Bank of India, Noorbaug, Mumbai-400009, Maharashtra, India
  Ph: 022-66661880/89 e-mail: mumbai@cbspd.com

Representatives

- Hyderabad 0-9885175004
- Jharkhand 0-9811541605
- Nagpur 0-9421945513
- Patna 0-9334159340
- Pune 0-9923910676
- Uttarakhand 0-9716462459

Printed at Chaman Offset, Delhi, India

Certificate

Student's Name Mr. / Ms. ______________________________

Class ______________________ *Roll No.* ______________________

Subject Pharmaceutical Analysis

This is to certify that experiments, written in the index, have been performed by the student, are satisfactory.

Grade..................

Name and signature of teacher

College stamp

Date ....

Preface

It gives us immense pleasure in writing this book *A Practical Approach to* ***Pharmaceutical Analysis***. A large number of theory books on 'instrumental analysis' have been published but practical books are not available in the market. We, therefore, felt that there was a great need to have a good book based on instrumental methods of analysis with practical approach, following both experimental as well as manual presentation. This book is designed keeping in view the syllabi of various universities in India and abroad. Viewing all aspects, the book starts with spectrophotometric analysis and covers various aspects of flame photometry, potentiometric titrations, fluorimetry, polarimetry, conductometric titration, refractometry, nepheloturbidimetry, chromatography (thin layer chromatography, paper chromatography, high performance liquid chromatography and high performance thin layer chromatography), interpretations of infrared spectras and mass spectras, miscellaneous methods including Karl Fischer titration and Kjeldahl's method.

A special emphasis has been given on the interpretations of infrared spectras and mass spectras, Karl Fischer titration and Kjeldahl's method. This book has been designed to serve as a ready-reckoner both for the students as well as the teachers, with a unique feature that the students can write their observations and calculations directly without wasting their valuable time. We hope this book will be useful to all undergraduate as well as postgraduate students.

We feel privileged to express our deep sense of gratitude to every one who has helped us at each and every step from inception to the publication of this book. Comments and suggestions on the content and approach of the book from all readers will be highly appreciated for making further improvement in the book.

Authors

Rajesh Kumar Nema

S. N. Meyyanathan

Chandra Shekhar Sharma

Mahesh Verma

C.S. Bhan

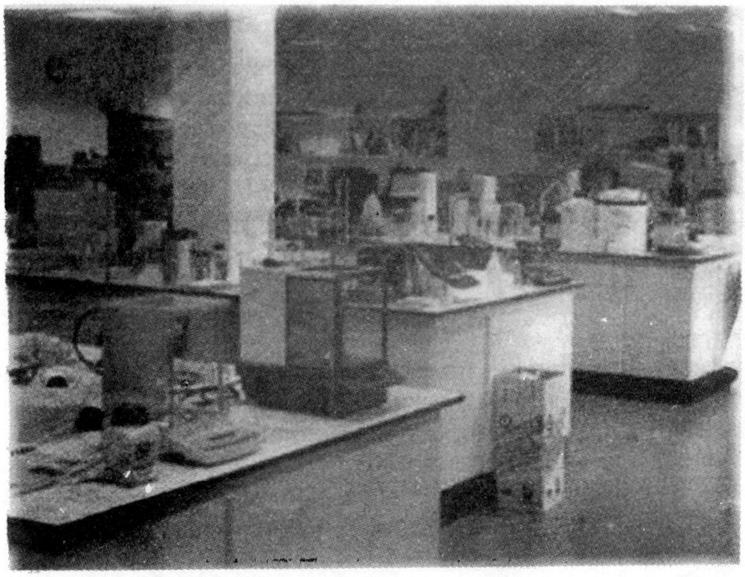

The Authors

RAJESH KUMAR NEMA

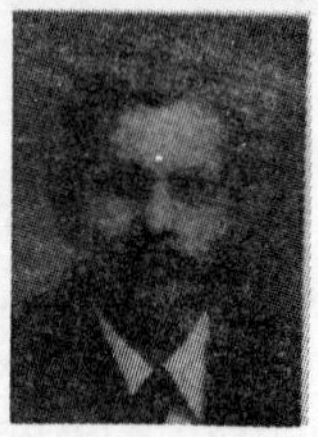

is currently Director, SD College of Pharmacy, Muzaffarnagar (UP), and has worked as Acting Principal, BNPG College of Pharmacy, Udaipur, for two years. He is an eminent teacher of pharmaceutical chemistry with more than 20 years of experience including teaching to postgraduate students for more than 6 years. Prof. Nema earned his B Pharm and M Pharm from Dr. HS Gaur Vishwavidyalya, Sagar and PhD from Mohan Lal Sukhadia University, Udaipur. He is elected as President, Association of Pharmaceutical Teachers of India (Rajasthan State Branch). Four candidates have registered for PhD programme under his supervision and he is a approved referee for assessment of PhD thesis and as an external examiner by various universities. He has authored several books and book chapters, published 20 research papers and 40 review articles in journals of national and international repute, and has attended various conferences. His fields of research interest are development of analytical methods, NDDS, and ocular and cosmetic products. He is a life member of IPA, ISTE, IHPA, APTI, IPGA.

S. N. MEYYANATHAN

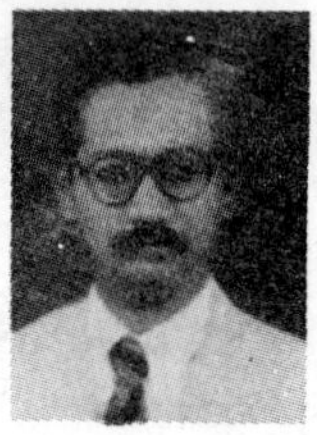

is presently Professor and Head, Department of Pharmaceutical Analysis, JSS College of Pharmacy, Ooty (Tamilnadu). He has 17 years of teaching experience and has published 39 research papers in various national and international journals of repute. He has guided 21 M Pharm and 4 PhD students. He has attended various national and international conferences. He is the life member of APTI and IPA, and is vice president of IPA (Nilgiri branch). Recently he has received a grant from AICTE, New Delhi, under research promotion scheme. His patent was published in drug synthesis.

CHANDRA SHEKHAR SHARMA

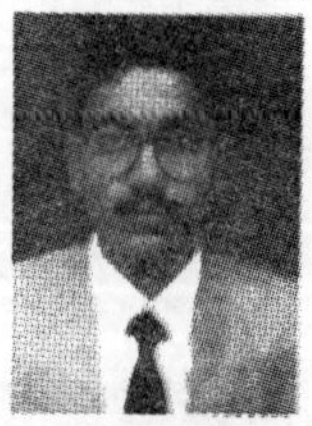

is presently Assistant Professor, Department of Pharmaceutical Chemistry, B N College of Pharmacy, Udaipur (Rajasthan). He completed his B Pharm from B N College of Pharmacy, Udaipur (Rajasthan), and M Pharm in pharmaceutical chemistry from JSS College of Pharmacy, Ooty (Tamilnadu). He has 3 years of teaching experience and has published 4 research papers in national and international journals. He has guided 13 B Pharm students.

MAHESH VERMA

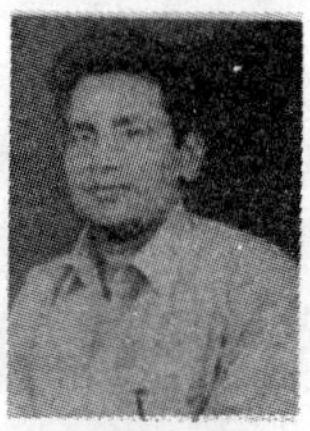

is presently on the Faculty of Pharmacy, Integral University, Lucknow (UP). He is a pharmacy graduate from Barkatullah University, Bhopal, and completed M Pharm in pharmaceutical chemistry from School of Pharmaceutical Sciences, RGPV, Bhopal. He has published various research papers in national and international conferences. He is a life member of APTI, ISTE and is a member of FIP, Netherland. He has participated in many national and international conferences, symposia and workshops.

PROF. C. S. BHAN

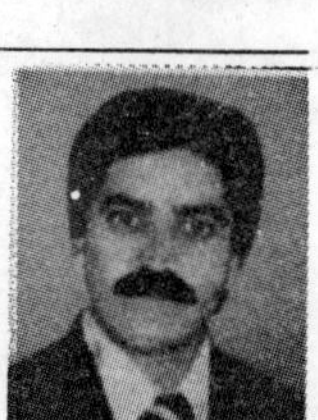

is presently Principal, MGCPS, Jaipur. He has specialisation in pharmaceutical chemistry with a teaching experience of 17 years. He has held a number of administrative positions as HoD/ Principal in a number of pharmacy institutions of Rajasthan. He is a life member of APTI and IHPA and has attended a number of conferences at national level.

Contents

EXPERIMENTS

EXPERIMENTS

EXPERIMENTS

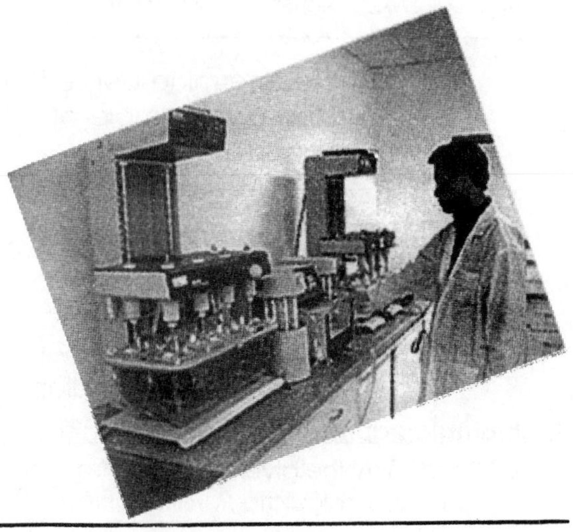

INDEX OF EXPERIMENTS

Date	Exp. No.	Topic	Page No.	Remarks
	1.1.	To determine the λ_{max} of Potassium Permanganate.		
	1.2.	To determine the percentage purity of given sample of Paracetamol by Spectroscopy.		
	1.3.	To perform the assay of Paracetamol tablet using calibration curve method.		
	1.4.	To determine the percentage purity of given sample of Isoniazid by Spectroscopy.		
	1.5.	To carry out the analysis of Diclofenac sodium and Paracetamol in combined dosage form.		
	1.6.	To study the effect of solvents upon the absorption spectrum of Griseofulvin.		
	1.7.	To find out percentage purity of Diltiazem HCl tablet I.P. by calibration curve method.		
	1.8.	To find out λ_{max} of Diltiazem HCl in different solvents.		
	1.9.	To determine percentage purity of the given sample of Chloramphenicol capsules I.P.		
	1.10.	To determine the percentage purity of given sample of Furosemide injection I.P.		
	1.11.	To determine the percentage purity of given sample of Allopurinol tablets I.P.		

Contd.

Contd.

Date	Exp. No.	Topic	Page No.	Remarks
	5.4.	To find out the percentage of glucose content in the marketed product of Oral Rehydration Salt (ORS).		
	6.1.	To determine the end-point and normality of given acid by conductometric titration.		
	6.2.	To carry out the conductometric titration of mixture of acids (0.1N HCl + 0.1N CH_3COOH) vs. strong base (1N NaOH)		
	7.1.	To find out the refractive indices of different liquids (Benzene, Glycerin and Water) by Abbes refractometer.		
	7.2.	To find out the molar refraction of benzene by abbe's refractometer and also confirm the structure of benzene.		
	7.3.	To find out the Concentration of unknown sample of glycerin by refractometry.		
	8.1.	To perform the limit test for chloride in the given solution by using nephloturbidimetry.		
	8.2.	To perform the limit test for sulphate in the given solution by using nephloturbidimetry.		
	9.1.	To identify the given sample of amino acid with the help of thin layer chromatography and also calculate R_f value of individual amino acids.		
	9.2.	To identify the given drug amongst the paracetamol, aspirin and caffeine citrate with the help of thin layer chromatography and calculate its R_f value.		

Contd.

Spectrophotometric Analysis

1

INTRODUCTION

Absorption spectrophotometry is an oldest method for quantitative analysis and structural elucidation. This is mainly concerned with the following regions of the spectrum — ultraviolet 100–400 nm, visible 400–800 nm and colorimetry. Colorimetry is concerned with the visible region of the spectrum. The instruments applied for measuring the absorption or emission of radiant energy from object are called by various names, such as

- Photometers,
- Colorimeters and
- Spectrophotometers.

Photometer. An instrument measures the ratio, or some functions of two, of the radiant power of two electromagnetic beams. Filters are used to isolate a narrow wavelength region and a photocell or phototube to measure the intensity of the radiation.

Colorimeter. Any instrument used for measuring absorption in the visible region is generally called a colorimeter. Some commercial filter photometers are called colorimeters.

Spectrophotometer. An instrument measures the ratio, or a function of two, of the radiant power of two electromagnetic beams over a large wavelength region. In this instrument is used monochromator instead of a filter. In addition, sensitive detectors like photomultipliers are used.

Theory of Spectrophotometric Analysis

Instrumentation

All photometers, colorimeters and spectrophotometers have the following basic components:

(*a*) Source
(*b*) Filter and monochromator
(*c*) Sample cell
(*d*) Detector

Laws Governing Absorption of Radiation

Many compounds absorb ultraviolet (UV) or visible light. The diagram below shows a beam of monochromatic radiation of radiant power P_0, directed at a sample solution.

Absorption takes place and the beam of radiation leaving the sample has radiant power P.

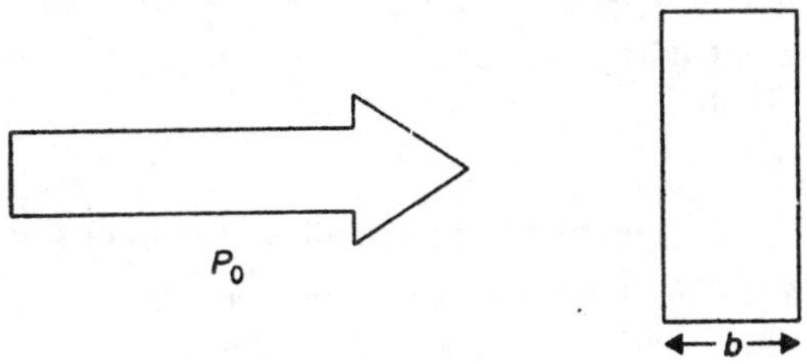

The amount of radiation absorbed may be measured in a number of ways:

Transmittance, $T = P/P_0$

% Transmittance, $\%T = 100\,T$

Absorbance,

$$A = \log_{10} P_0/P$$
$$A = \log_{10} 1/T$$
$$A = \log_{10} 100/\%T$$
$$A = 2 - \log_{10} \%T$$

The last equation, $A = 2 - \log_{10} \%T$, is worth remembering because it allows you to easily calculate absorbance from percentage transmittance data.

The relationship between absorbance and transmittance is illustrated in the following diagram:

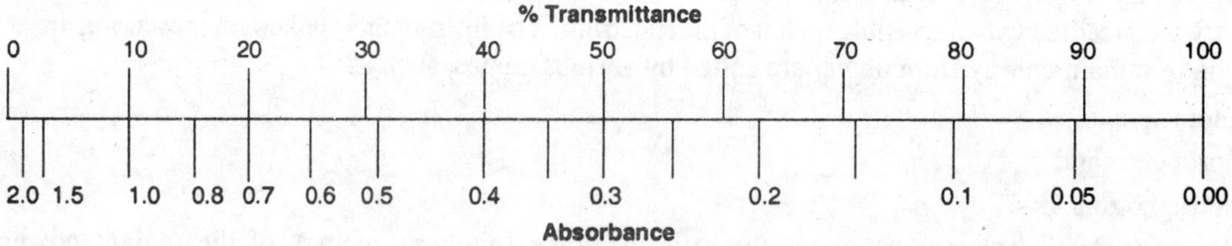

So, if all the light passes through a solution without any absorption, then absorbance is zero, and percent transmittance is 100%. If all the light is absorbed, then percent transmittance is zero, and absorption is infinite.

Laws Governing Absorption of Radiation

When light is incident upon a homogenous medium, a part of the incident light is reflected, a part is absorbed by the medium and the reminder is allowed to transmit as such. So

$$I_0 = I_a + I_r + I_t \tag{1}$$

where

I_0 = incident light

I_a = part of light absorbed

I_r = part of incident light reflected

I_t = part of light transmit as such

If a comparison cell is used, the value of I_r, which is very small, can be eliminated for air-glass interfaces. Under this condition, eq. (1) becomes as

$$I_0 = I_a + I_t \tag{2}$$

LAMBERT'S LAW

This law states that "when a beam of light is allowed to pass through a transparent medium, the rate of decrease of intensity with the thickness of medium is directly proportional to the intensity of the light."

Mathematically, it can be represented as

$$I_t = I_0\, e^{-kt} \tag{3}$$

Where I_0 denotes the intensity of the incident light, I_t denotes the intensity of the transmitted light and k is a constant which depends upon the wavelength and absorbing medium used.

BEER'S LAW

This law states that the intensity of a beam of monochromatic light decreases exponentially with the increase in concentration of the absorbing substance arithmetically. Mathematically, it can be represented as

$$I_t = I_0 e^{-k'c}$$

or $$I_t = I_0 10^{-0.4343\,k'c}$$

or $$I_t = I_0 10^{-K'c} \quad (4)$$

Where k' and K' are constants and c is the concentration of the absorbing substance.

On combining equation (3) and (4), we get

$$I_t = I_0 10^{-act}$$

or $$\log I_0/I_t = act \quad (5)$$

Equation (5) is termed as mathematical statement of **Beer–Lambert law**. This is also the fundamental equation of colorimetry and spectrophotometry.

Deviation from Beer's Law

From Beer's law it follows that if we plot absorbance A against concentration, a straight line passing through the origin should be obtained. But there is usually a deviation from a linear relationship between concentration and absorbance and an apparent failure of Beer's law may ensure. Deviation from the law are reported as positive or negative, according to whether the curve is concave upward or concave downward.

Factors:

1. Deviation may occur due to presence of impurities that fluorescence absorb at the absorption wavelength.
2. If monochromatic light is not used.
3. If width of slit is not proper, therefore it allows undesirable radiations to fall on the detector.

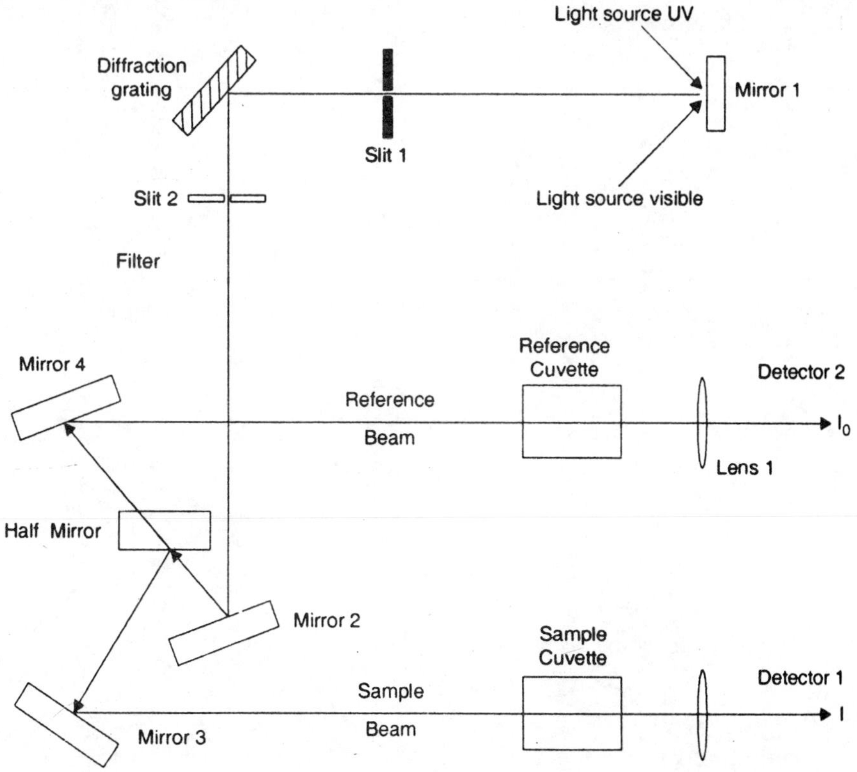

Fig. Double beam spectrophotometer

4. If the solution species undergoes polymerization, so deviation may occur. Example, benzyl alcohol in carbon tetrachloride in high concentration exists in polymeric form, $[(C_6H_5CH_2OH)_4]$, dissociation of this polymer increases with dilution. Due to this change, absorbance will change.
5. Beer's law cannot be applied to suspensions, but latter can be estimated colorimetrically after preparing a reference curve with known concentration.
6. Deviation may also occur, if the coloured solute ionizes, dissociates or associates in solution. Example, benzyl alcohol in chloroform exists in a polymeric equilibrium $4C_6H_5CH_2OH \longleftrightarrow (C_6H_5CH_2OH)_4$.
7. If concentration change causes significant alterations in the refractive index of a solution, deviation from Beer's law is observed.
8. Deviation may occur, in case the absorbing material is coagulated into small number of large units. Because coagulated particles will cause turbidity that is scattering of beam of radiation (↑ or ↓ in absorption).

EXPERIMENT 1.1 A

Date ______________

COLORIMETRY

AIM

To determine the λ_{max} of potassium permanganate.

PRINCIPLE

The principle behind the determination of λ_{max} for any coloured substance (e.g. $KMnO_4$) is that the coloured substance absorbs maximum radiation at a particular wavelength in the visible region, which ranges from 400–800 nm. These coloured substances absorb the radiation in different manner depending upon the wavelengths used.

This unique property of maximum absorption at a particular wavelength is known as λ_{max} and is useful for identification of that particular substance. The λ_{max} is usually not affected by the concentration used.

Mol. Formula: $KMnO_4$ **Mol. Wt.:** 158.03

Solubility: Soluble in cold water; freely soluble in boiling water.

Category: Antiseptic.

ASSAY

Weigh accurately about 0.3 g, dissolve in sufficient water to produce 100 ml. To 20 ml add 20 ml of water, 1 g of potassium iodide and 10 ml of 2M hydrochloric acid and titrate the liberated iodine with 0.1M sodium thiosulphate using starch solution, added towards the end of the titration as indicator. Each ml of 0.1M sodium thiosulphate is equivalent to 0.003160 g of $KMnO_4$.

PROCEDURE

1. Weigh accurately 100 mg of $KMnO_4$ and dissolve in 30 ml distilled water in a volumetric flask.
2. Make the volume up to 100 ml with distilled water.
3. Take 10 ml of above solution and dilute to 100 ml with distilled water.
4. Now finally take 4 ml of above solution and diluted to 10 ml with distilled water in order to get the resulting solution (40 μg/ml).
5. Switch on the colorimeter and allow to stabilize for 15 minutes.
6. Set the absorbance at zero by using distilled water as the blank.
7. Now set 100% transmittance by distilled water.
8. Take the absorbance of the resulting solution at different wavelengths.
9. Plot the graph between wavelength *vs.* observed absorbance.

Note: The wavelength selection should be in order to get maximum absorption.

OBSERVATIONS

S. No.	Wavelength (nm)	Absorbance
1.	400 nm	0.07
2.	450 nm	0.10
3.	500 nm	0.21

(Contd.)

S. No.	Wavelength (nm)	Absorbance
4.	550 nm	0.36
5.	555 nm	0.38
6.	560 nm	0.35
7.	575 nm	0.23
8.	600 nm	0.05
9.	650 nm	0.04
10.	700 nm	0.02

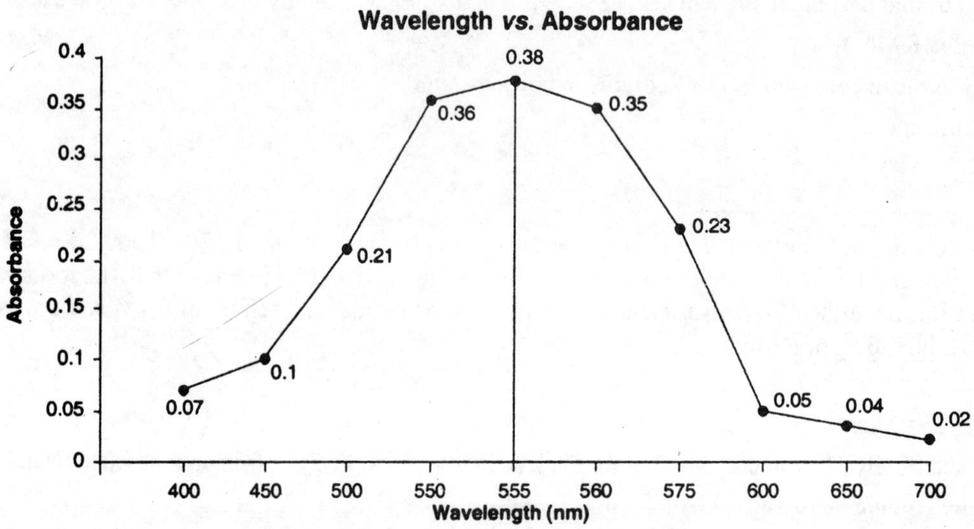

DISCUSSION

From the graph, the maximum absorbance (0.38) is observed at 555 nm wavelength.

RESULT

The λ_{max} of potassium permanganate was found to be 555 nm.

EXPERIMENT 1.1B

Date ____________

COLORIMETRY

(Manual)

AIM

To determine the λ_{max} of potassium permanganate.

PROCEDURE

1. Weigh accurately 100 mg of $KMnO_4$ and dissolve in 30 ml distilled water in a volumetric flask.
2. Make the volume up to 100 ml with distilled water.
3. Take 10 ml of above solution and dilute to 100 ml with distilled water.
4. Now finally take 4 ml of above solution and dilute to 10 ml with distilled water in order to get the resulting solution (40 μg/ml).
5. Switch on the colorimeter and allow to stabilize for 15 minutes.
6. Set the absorbance at zero by using distilled water as the blank.
7. Now set 100% transmittance by distilled water.
8. Take the absorbance of the resulting solution at different wavelengths.
9. Plot the graph between wavelength *vs.* observed absorbance.

Note: The wavelength selection should be in order to get maximum absorption.

OBSERVATIONS

S. No.	Wavelength (nm)	Absorbance
1.	400 nm	
2.	450 nm	
3.	500 nm	
4.	550 nm	
5.	555 nm	
6.	560 nm	
7.	575 nm	
8.	600 nm	
9.	650 nm	
10.	700 nm	

DISCUSSION

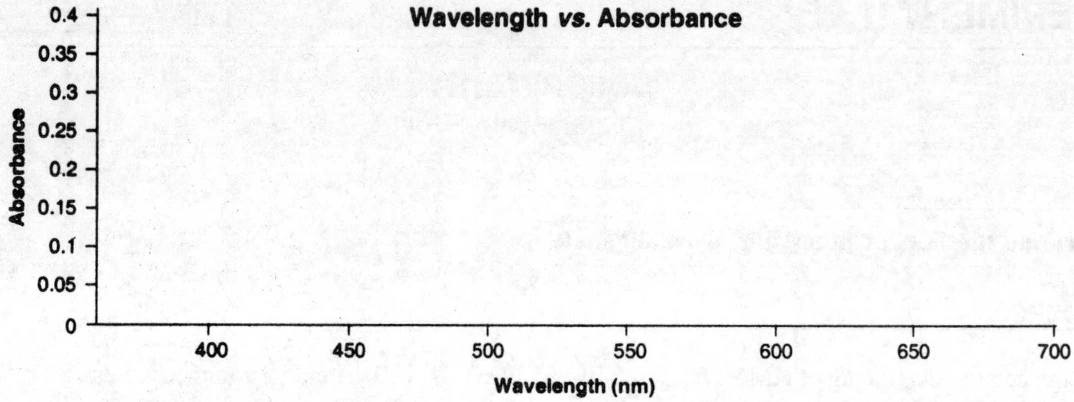

From the graph, the maximum absorbance (________) is observed at ________ nm wavelength.

RESULT

The λ_{max} of potassium permanganate was found to be ________ nm.

EXPERIMENT 1.2A

Date ______________

ASSAY OF PARACETAMOL TABLETS I.P.

AIM

To determine the percentage purity of given sample of paracetamol by spectroscopy.

ACETAMINOPHEN

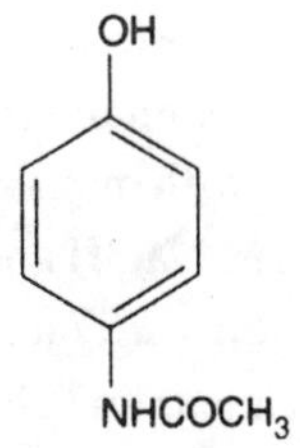

Paracetamol is 4-hydroxyacetanilide

Mol. Formula: $C_8H_9NO_2$ **Mol.Wt.:** 151.16

SOLUBILITY

Freely soluble in ethanol (95%) and in acetone; sparingly soluble in water; very slightly soluble in dichloromethane and in ether.

CATEGORY

Analgesic; antipyretic.

ASSAY

Weigh accurately about 0.5 g, dissolve in a mixture of 10 ml of water and 50 ml of 1 M sulphuric acid. Boil under reflux condenser for 1 hour, cool and dilute to 100 ml with water. To 20 ml of the solution add 40 ml of water, 40 g of water in the form of ice, 15 ml of 2 M hydrochloric acid and 0.1 ml of ferroin solution and titrate with 0.1M ceric ammonium sulphate until a yellow colour is produced. Perform a blank determination and make any necessary correction. Each ml of 0.1 M cerric ammonium sulphate is equivalent to 0.00756 g of $C_8H_9NO_2$.

USES

Paracetamol is used in pain including dysmenorrhoea, headache; pain relief in osteoarthritis and soft tissue lesions; pyrexia including post-immunization pyrexia; also acute migraine attack. **Paracetamol** is similar in analgesic and antipyretic efficacy to acetylsalicylic acid. It is used for mild to moderate pain including headache and acute migraine attacks and for reducing fever, including post-immunization pyrexia. Paracetamol is particularly useful in patients in whom salicylates or other NSAIDs are contraindicated, such as asthmatics and those with a history of peptic ulcer, or for children under the age of 12 years in whom salicylates are contraindicated because of the risk of Reye syndrome. It is generally preferred to acetylsalicylic acid, particularly in the elderly, because it is less irritant to the stomach. Unlike acetylsalicylic acid and other NSAIDs. Paracetamol has little anti-inflammatory activity which limits its usefulness for long-term treatment of pain associated with inflammation; however it is useful in the management of osteoarthritis, a condition with only a small inflammatory component. In normal doses adverse effects are rare, but over dosage with a single dose of 10–15 g is particularly dangerous because it may cause hepatocellular necrosis and, less frequently, renal tubular necrosis.

Paracetamol is insoluble in water, so NaOH is used to solubilize the tablet and since paracetamol contains OH groups. As auxochrome which modifies the absorption of chromophore. As a result paracetamol absorbs in UV region at **257** nm. $E^{1\%}_{1cm}$ (Molecular extinct coefficient) of paracetamol at 257 nm is 715.

PROCEDURE

1. Weigh and powder 20 tablets with the help of mortar and pestle.
2. Weigh accurately a quantity of the powdered tablets equivalent to 0.15 gm of paracetamol.
3. Add 50 ml of 0.1M NaOH and dilute to 100 ml with distilled water.
4. Shake for 15 min. and add sufficient distilled water to produce 200 ml.
5. Mix well and filter the resulting solution with Whatmann filter paper.
6. Take 10 ml of this solution and dilute to 100 ml with distilled water.
7. To 10 ml of resulting solution, add 10 ml of 0.1M NaOH and dilute to 100 ml with distilled water and mix well.
8. Measure the absorbance of the resulting solution at 257 nm against blank solution.

Note: The solution ready for absorbance should be clear and should not contain any particle.

OBSERVATIONS

1. Weight variation test

S. No.	Wt. of tablets (gm)	S. No.	Wt. of tablets (gm)
1	0.620	11	0.620
2	0.610	12	0.610
3	0.617	13	0.617
4	0.620	14	0.620
5	0.610	15	0.610
6	0.617	16	0.617
7	0.619	17	0.619
8	0.620	18	0.620
9	0.610	19	0.610
10	0.617	20	0.617
		Average weight (gm)	0.618

2. Absorbance (A) = 0.533.

CALCULATIONS

1. Label claim of given tablet = 0.500 gm.
2. Weight of 20 tablets = 12.36 gm.
3. Average weight of tablets = 0.618 gm.
   0.618 gm of powder = 0.500 gm of PCM.

$\therefore$ x gm of powder = 0.15 gm of PCM.

$$\therefore\ x = \frac{0.15 \times 0.618}{0.500} = \mathbf{0.185\ gm}$$

$$\textbf{\% Dilution Factor} = \frac{0.185}{200} \times \frac{10}{100} \times \frac{10}{100} \times 100$$

$$= 0.000925\%\ \text{w/v.}$$

FORMULA

$$\%\ \text{purity} = \frac{A}{E^{1\%}_{1\,cm}} \times \frac{\text{Avg. wt.}}{\text{L.C.}} \times \frac{100}{\text{Dil. Factor}}$$

$$= \frac{0.533}{715} \times \frac{0.618}{0.500} \times \frac{100}{0.000925}$$

$$= \mathbf{99.60\%\ w/w.}$$

RESULT

The percentage purity of given sample of 0.500 gm of Paracetamol tablets I.P. was found to be 99.61% w/w.

EXPERIMENT 1.2B

Date ____________

ASSAY OF PARACETAMOL TABLETS I.P.
(Manual)

AIM

To determine the percentage purity of given sample of paracetamol.

PROCEDURE

1. Weigh and powder 20 tablets with the help of mortar and pestle.
2. Weigh accurately a quantity of the powdered tablets equivalent to 0.15 gm of Paracetamol.
3. Add 50 ml of 0.1M NaOH and dilute to 100 ml with distilled water.
4. Shake for 15 minute and add sufficient distilled water to produce 200 ml.
5. Mix well and filter the resulting solution with Whatmann filter paper.
6. Take 10 ml of this solution and dilute to 100 ml with distilled water.
7. To 10 ml of resulting solution, add 10 ml of 0.1M NaOH and dilute to 100 ml with distilled water and mix well.
8. Measure the absorbance of the resulting solution at 257 nm against blank solution.

Note: The solution ready for absorbance should be clear and should not contain any particle.

OBSERVATIONS

1. Weight variation test

S. No.	Wt. of tablets (gm)	S. No.	Wt. of tablets (gm)
1		11	
2		12	
3		13	
4		14	
5		15	
6		16	
7		17	
8		18	
9		19	
10		20	
		Average weight (gm)	

2. Absorbance (A) =

CALCULATIONS

1. Label claim of given tablet = ________
2. Weight of 20 tablets = ________
3. Average weight of tablets = ________

________gm of powder ≡ ________ gm of PCM.

∴ x gm of powder ≡ ________ gm of PCM.

∴ X = ________

% Dilution Factor = ________

= ________ % w/v.

FORMULA

$$\% \text{ purity} = \frac{E}{E_{cm}^{1\%}} \times \frac{\text{Avg. wt.}}{\text{L.C.}} \times \frac{100}{\text{Dil. Factor}}$$

= ________

= ________ **% w/w.**

RESULT

The percentage purity of given sample of 0.500 gm of Paracetamol tablets I.P. was found be ________% w/w.

EXPERIMENT 1.3 A

Date ____________

ASSAY OF PARACETAMOL TABLETS I.P.

AIM

To perform the assay of paracetamol tablet using calibration curve method.

PRINCIPLE

In calibration curve method, a calibration curve is plotted both concentration *vs.* absorbance value of more than five standard dilutions. A straight line is drawn in such a manner that it should pass maximum number of points. This method is called as **Line of Best Fit.** This is not necessary that the line should pass through the origin.

PROCEDURE

1. **Preparation of standard dilutions**
   (*a*) Weigh accurately 100 mg of Paracetamol pure powdered drug and add 50 ml of 0.1M NaOH and dilute to 100 ml with distilled water.
   (*b*) Take 10 ml of above solution and dilute up to 100 ml with distilled water.
   (*c*) Prepare 6 standard dilutions from above stock solution by diluting 0.5 ml, 1.0 ml, 1.5 ml, 2.0 ml, 2.5 ml and 3.0 ml to 10 ml with 0.1M NaOH.
   (*d*) Run these 6 standard dilutions of 5 μg/ml, 10 μg/ml, 15 μg/ml, 20 μg/ml, 25 μg/ml and 30 μg/ml concentration for absorbance against blank.
   (*e*) Plot calibration curve between absorbance *vs.* concentration at 257 nm.
   (*f*) Find out the equation of line.
2. **Preparation of sample solution (tablets)**
   (*a*) Weigh and powder 20 tablets with the help of mortar and pestle.
   (*b*) Weigh accurately a quantity of the powdered tablets equivalent to 0.15 gm of Paracetamol.
   (*c*) Add 50 ml of 0.1M NaOH and dilute to 100 ml with distilled water.
   (*d*) Shake for 15 min. and add sufficient distilled water to produce 200 ml.
   (*e*) Mix well and filter the resulting solution with Whatmann filter paper.
   (*f*) Take 10 ml of this solution and dilute to 100 ml with distilled water.
   (*g*) To 10 ml of resulting solution, add 10 ml of 0.1M NaOH and dilute to 100 ml with distilled water and mix well.
   (*h*) Measure the absorbance of the resulting solution at 257 nm against blank solution.

   After observing the absorbance, calculate the consent by equation.

OBSERVATION

1. **Weight variation test**

S. No.	Wt. of tablets (gm)	S. No.	Wt. of tablets (gm)
1.	0.609	2.	0.616
3.	0.617	4.	0.619
5.	0.615	6.	0.616
7.	0.617	8.	0.618

(Contd.)

S. No.	Wt. of tablets (gm)	S. No.	Wt. of tablets (gm)
9.	0.619	10.	0.611
11.	0.621	12.	0.622
13.	0.623	14.	0.624
15.	0.625	16.	0.628
17.	0.627	18.	0.615
19.	0.611	20.	0.605
	Average weight (gm)		**0.61875**

2. Absorbance of standard dilutions

S. No.	Concentration of Paracetamol (μg /ml)	Absorbance
1.	5.00	0.457
2.	10.00	0.768
3.	15.00	1.045
4.	20.00	1.568
5.	25.00	1.865
6.	30.00	2.264
7.	**Sample**	0.595

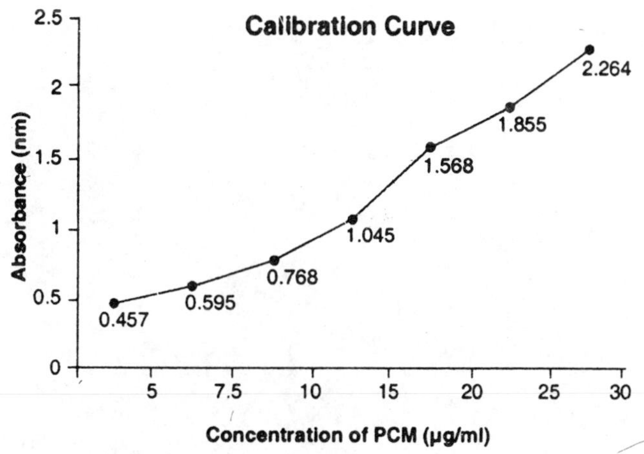

3. Absorbance of sample solution (tablet) (A) = 0.595

150 mg diluted to 200 ml (0.1M NaOH + water) = 0.75 mg/ml

10 ml of 0.75 mg/ml diluted to 100 ml (distilled water) = 0.075 mg/ml

Again 10 ml of 0.075 mg/ml diluted to 100 ml (distilled water) = 0.0075 mg/ml

0.0075 mg/ml = 7.5 μg /ml (concentration of test dilution)

CALCULATIONS

$$Y = mx + c$$

where, $m = 0.0743$

$c = 0.0373$ (from graphs)

$$Y = 0.0743\,x + 0.0373$$

$\because$ Y = absorbance of the sample solution (tablet), i.e. **0.595**

$$\therefore \quad 0.595 = 0.0743\,x + 0.0373$$

$$\therefore \quad x = \frac{0.595 - 0.0373}{0.0743}$$

$$\therefore \quad x = \mathbf{7.506\ \mu g/ml.}$$

As the concentration of sample solution (tablet) is 7.5 mg/ml (As per label claim)

$$\therefore \quad \%\text{ label claim} = \frac{\text{Concentration of sample practically}}{\text{Concentration of sample found theoretically}} \times 100$$

$$= \frac{7.506}{7.5} \times 100$$

$$= 100.08\ \%\ \text{w/w}$$

RESULT

The percentage purity of given sample of 500 mg Paracetamol tablet by calibration curve method was found to be 100.08% w/w.

EXPERIMENT 1.3 B

Date ______________

ASSAY OF PARACETAMOL TABLETS I.P.

(Manual)

AIM

To perform the assay of paracetamol tablet using calibration curve method.

PROCEDURE

1. **Preparation of standard dilutions**
   (*a*) Weigh accurately 100 mg of Paracetamol pure powdered drug and add 50 ml of 0.1M NaOH and dilute to 100 ml with distilled water.
   (*b*) Take 10 ml of above solution and dilute up to 100 ml with distilled water.
   (*c*) Prepare 6 standard dilutions from above stock solution by diluting 0.5 ml, 1.0 ml, 1.5 ml, 2.0 ml, 2.5 ml and 3.0 ml to 10 ml with 0.1M NaOH.
   (*d*) Run these 6 standard dilutions of 5 μg/ml, 10 μg/ml, 15 μg/ml, 20 μg/ml, 25 μg/ml and 30 μg/ml concentration for absorbance against blank.
   (*e*) Plot calibration curve between absorbance *vs.* concentration at 257 nm.
   (*f*) Find out the equation of line.
2. **Preparation of sample solution (tablets)**
   (*a*) Weigh and powder 20 tablets with the help of mortar and pestle.
   (*b*) Weigh accurately a quantity of the powdered tablets equivalent to 0.15 gm of Paracetamol.
   (*c*) Add 50 ml of 0.1M NaOH and dilute to 100 ml with distilled water.
   (*d*) Shake for 15 min. and add sufficient distilled water to produce 200 ml.
   (*e*) Mix well and filter the resulting solution with Whatmann filter paper.
   (*f*) Take 10 ml of this solution and dilute to 100 ml with distilled water.
   (*g*) To 10 ml of resulting solution, add 10 ml of 0.1M NaOH and dilute to 100 ml with distilled water and mix well.
   (*h*) Measure the absorbance of the resulting solution at 257 nm against blank solution.

   After observing the absorbance, calculate the consent by equation.

OBSERVATION

1. **Weight variation test**

S. No.	Wt. of tablets (gm)	S. No.	Wt. of tablets (gm)
1.		11.	
2.		12.	
3.		13.	
4.		14.	
5.		15.	
6.		16.	
7.		17.	
8.		18.	
9.		19.	
10.		20.	
	Average weight (gm)		

2. Absorbance of standard dilutions

S. No.	Concentration of Paracetamol (µg /ml)	Absorbance
1.	5.00	
2.	10.00	
3.	15.00	
4.	20.00	
5.	25.00	
6.	30.00	
7.	Sample	

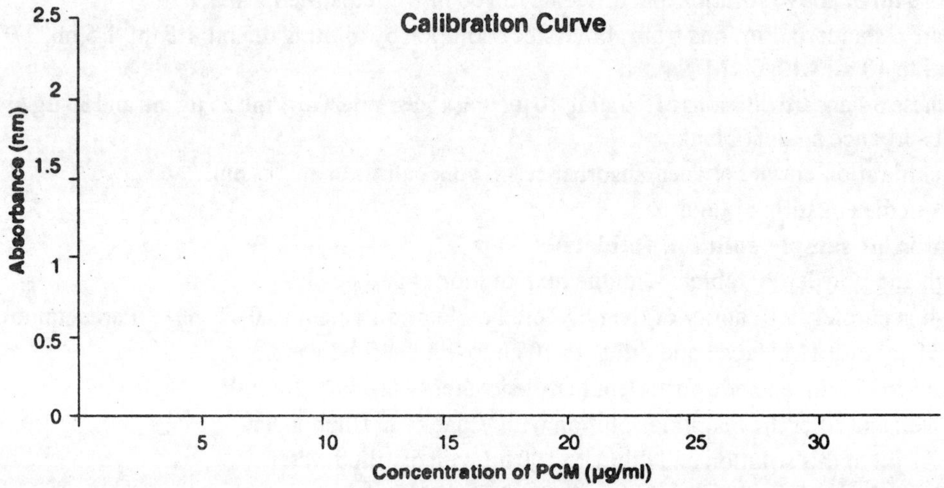

3. Absorbance of sample solution (tablet) (A) = ______
150 mg diluted to 200 ml (0.1M NaOH + water) = ______ mg/ml
10 ml of 0.75 mg/ml diluted to 100 ml (distilled water) = ______ mg/ml
Again 10 ml of 0.075 mg/ml diluted to 100 ml (distilled water) = ______ mg/ml
______ **mg/ml =** ______ µg /ml (concentration of test dilution)

CALCULATIONS

$$Y = mx + c$$

where, m = ______
c = ______ (from graph)
$\because$ Y = absorbance of the sample solution (tablet) i.e. ______

$\therefore$ ______ = ______ x + ______

$$\therefore \quad x = \frac{\_\_\_\_\_\_ - \_\_\_\_\_\_}{\_\_\_\_\_\_}$$

$\therefore \quad x =$ ________ µg/ml.

As the concentration of sample solution (tablet) is ______ mg/ml (As per label claim)

$$\therefore \quad \text{\% label claim} = \frac{\text{Concentration of sample practically}}{\text{Concentration of sample found theoretically}} \times 100$$

= ________ × 100

= ________ % w/w

RESULT

The percentage purity of given sample of 500 mg Paracetamol tablet by calibration curve method was found to be ________% w/w.

EXPERIMENT 1.4 A

Date ____________

ASSAY OF ISONIAZID TABLETS

AIM

To determine the percentage purity of given sample of isoniazid by spectroscopy.

PRINCIPLE

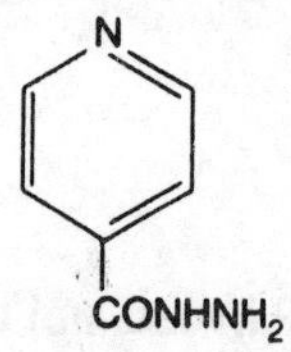

Mol. Formula: $C_6H_7N_3O$ **Mol. Wt.:** 137.14

Isoniazid is isonicotinohydrazide.

SOLUBILITY

Freely soluble in water; sparingly soluble in ethanol (95%); slightly soluble in chloroform; very slightly soluble in ether.

CATEGORY

Antitubercular.

ASSAY

Weigh accurately about 0.25 g, dissolve in sufficient water to produce 100 ml. To 20 ml of the resulting solution add 100 ml of water, 20 ml of hydrochloric acid and 0.2 g of potassium bromide and titrate slowly with continuous shaking with 0.0167M potassium bromate using 0.05 ml of methyl red solution as indicator, until the red colour disappears.

Each ml of 0.0167M potassium bromate is equivalent to 0.003429 g of $C_6H_7N_3O$.

λ_{max} = 266 nm.

The $E^{1\%}_{1cm}$ value of Isoniazid at 266 nm is **378.**

PROCEDURE

1. Weigh accurately 20 tablets and calculate average weight.
2. Powder the tablets with mortar and pestle.
3. Weigh accurately the powdered quantity equivalent to 0.100 gm of Isoniazid.
4. Extract the weighed quantity with 3 portions of 25 ml each of water.
5. Filter and collect the filtrate in 100 ml volumetric flash.
6. Wash the residue with 10 ml of water and filter the washing.
7. Dilute the solution to 100 ml with water so that the final concentration will reach at 10 µg/ml.
8. Take 10 ml of this solution and dilute to 100 ml with distilled water.
9. Again take 10 ml and dilute to 100 ml with distilled water to get 10 µg/ml concentration of the resulting solution.
10. Make sure that the solution do not contain any particle and run into the spectrophotometer for absorbance at 266 nm.

OBSERVATIONS

1. Weight variation test

S. No.	Wt. of tablets (gm)	S. No.	Wt. of tablets (gm)
1.	0.567	11.	0.569
2.	0.566	12.	0.563
3.	0.565	13.	0.564
4.	0.568	14.	0.568
5.	0.564	15.	0.566
6.	0.567	16.	0.563
7.	0.565	17.	0.569
8.	0.567	18.	0.568
9.	0.566	19.	0.564
10.	0.565	20.	0.565
	Average weight (gm)		0.566

2. Absorbance $A = 0.369$

CALCULATIONS

Label claim of given tablet = 0.300 gm

Weight of 20 tablets = 11.32 gm

Average weight of tablet = 0.566 gm

0.566 gm of powder ≡ 0.300 gm of INH

∴ x gm of powder ≡ 0.100 gm of INH

$$\therefore \quad x = \frac{0.566 \times 0.100}{0.300}$$

$$x = \mathbf{0.1887} \text{ gm of powder.}$$

Dilution Factor Calculation:

0.1887 gm of powder diluted to 100 ml = 0.001887 gm/ml

10 ml of this solution diluted to 100 ml = 0.0001887 gm/ml

Again 10 ml of this solution diluted to 100 ml = 0.00001887 gm/ml

0.00001887 gm/ml = 0.0018% w/v

FORMULA

$$\% \text{ purity} = \frac{A}{E^{1\%}_{1\text{cm}}} \times \frac{\text{Avg. wt.}}{\text{L.C.}} \times \frac{100}{\text{D.F.}}$$

$$= \frac{0.369}{378} \times \frac{0.566}{0.300} \times \frac{100}{0.0018} = \mathbf{102.31\% \text{ w/w}}$$

RESULT

The percentage purity of given sample Isoniazid tablet I.P. by Spectrophotometry was found to be **102.31% w/w.**

EXPERIMENT 1.4B

Date ________

ASSAY OF ISONIAZID TABLETS
(Manual)

AIM

To determine the percentage purity of given sample of isoniazid by spectroscopy.

GIVEN

$$\lambda_{max} = 266 \text{ nm.}$$

The $E^{1\%}_{1cm}$ value of Isoniazid at 266 nm is 378.

PROCEDURE

1. Weigh accurately 20 tablets and calculate average weight.
2. Powder the tablets with mortar and pestle.
3. Weigh accurately the powdered quantity equivalent to 0.100 gm of Isoniazid.
4. Extract the weighed quantity with 3 portions of 25 ml each of water.
5. Filter and collect the filtrate in 100 ml volumetric flash.
6. Wash the residue with 10 ml of water and filter the washing.
7. Dilute the solution to 100 ml with water so that the final concentration will reach at10 μg/ml.
8. Take 10 ml of this solution and dilute to 100 ml with distilled water.
9. Again take 10 ml and dilute to 100 ml with distilled water to get 10 μg/ml concentration of the resulting solution.
10. Make sure that the solution do not contain any particle and run into the spectrophotometer for absorbance at 266 nm.

OBSERVATIONS

1. Weight variation test

S. No.	Wt. of tablets (gm)	S. No.	Wt. of tablets (gm)
1.		11.	
2.		12.	
3.		13.	
4.		14.	
5.		15.	
6.		16.	
7.		17.	
8.		18.	
9.		19.	
10.		20.	
	Average weight (gm)		

2. Absorbance A = ________

CALCULATIONS

Label claim of given tablet = ________ gm

Weight of 20 tablets = ________ gm

Average weight of tablet = ________ gm

________ gm of powder ≡ 0.300 gm of INH

∴ x gm of powder ≡ 0.100 gm of INH

x = ________ gm of powder.

Dilution Factor Calculation

________ gm of powder diluted to 100 ml = ________ gm/ml

10 ml of this solution diluted to 100 ml = ________ gm/ml

Again 10 ml of this solution diluted to 100 ml = ________ gm/ml

________ gm/ml = ________ % w/v

FORMULA

$$\% \text{ purity} = \frac{A}{E^{1\%}_{1\text{cm}}} \times \frac{\text{Avg. wt.}}{\text{L.C.}} \times \frac{100}{\text{D.F.}}$$

= ________

= ________ % w/w

RESULT

The percentage purity of given sample Isoniazid tablet I.P. by Spectrophotometry was found to be ______ % w/w.

EXPERIMENT 1.5 A

Date ____________

ASSAY OF DICLOFENAC SODIUM AND PARACETAMOL

AIM

To carry out the analysis of diclofenac sodium and paracetamol in combined dosage form.

PRINCIPLE

There are several methods of multi component analysis depending upon various properties of individual component should meet certain conditions:

1. There should not be any chemical interaction between the components.
2. The solvent for extraction should be selective for one component and should not react with another component in the multi component mixture.
3. The individual component must show different absorption spectra. The various methods of multi component analysis are:
   (*a*) Assay by correcting the absorbance for the other substance
   (*b*) Solvent extraction method
   (*c*) Simultaneous multi component estimation methods
   (*d*) Assay using absorption ratio of the drugs.

The principle behind estimation of paracetamol and diclofenac solution in combined formulation is, the each component can be separated by solvent extraction methods, i.e. paracetamol can be extracted with 0.1N HCl solution and after filtration, the filtrate can be used for paracetamol estimation and the residue can be used for estimation of diclofenac sodium with the help of 0.1N NaOH.

The concentration of each component can be estimated by direct comparison method using standard solution of each with the formula.

$$C_2 = C_1 \times A_2/A_1 \text{ (derived from equation } A = \varepsilon Ct)$$

where,

C_1 and C_2 are the concentrations of standard and sample solution respectively

A_1 and A_2 are the absorbances of standard and sample solution respectively

ε = molecular extinction coefficient

t = path length

DICLOFENAC SODIUM

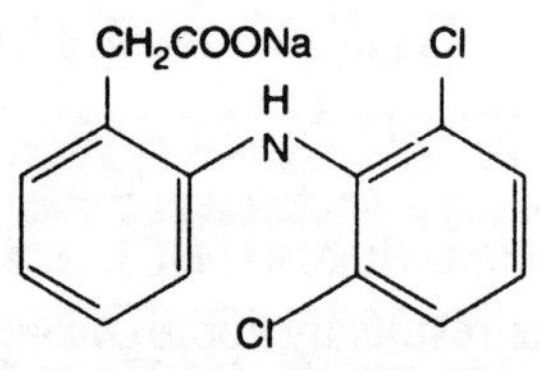

Mol. Formula: $C_{14}H_{10}Cl_2NNaO_2$ **Mol. Wt.:** 318.13

Diclofenac sodium is sodium 2-[(2, 6-dichlorophenyl)-amino] phenyl acetate.

Category: Analgesic; anti-inflammatory.

Description: White to slightly yellowish crystalline powder; slightly hygroscopic.

Solubility: Freely soluble in methanol; soluble in ethanol (95%); sparingly soluble in water and in glacial acetic acid; practically insoluble in ether, in chloroform and in toluene.

ASSAY

Weigh accurately about 0.2 g, dissolve in 50 ml of anhydrous glacial acetic acid and carry out the Method A as given in I.P. 1996 (Appendix 3.45) for non-aqueous titration, determining the end-point potentiometrically. Perform a blank determination and make any necessary correction. Each ml of 0.1M perchloric acid is equivalent to **0.03181 g of $C_{14}H_{10}Cl_2NNaO_2$.**

ACETAMINOPHEN (PARACETAMOL)

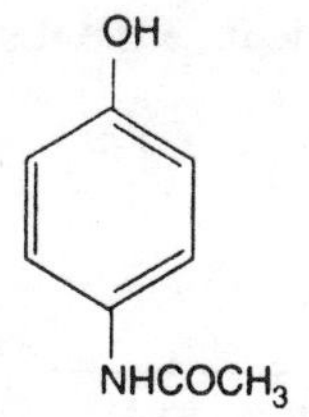

Mol. Formula: $C_8H_9NO_2$ **Mol. Wt.:** 151.16

Paracetamol is 4-hydroxyacetanilide.

Category: Analgesic; antipyretic.

Description: White crystals or white crystalline powder.

Solubility: Freely soluble in ethanol (95%) and in acetone; sparingly soluble in water; very slightly soluble in dichloromethane and in ether.

Assay: Weigh accurately about 0.5 g, dissolve in a mixture of 10 ml of water and 50 ml of 1M sulphuric acid. Boil under reflux condenser for 1 hour, cool and dilute to 100.0 ml with water. To 20.0 ml of the solution, add 40 ml of water, 40 g of water in the form of ice, 15 ml of 2M hydrochloric acid and 0.1 ml of ferroin solution and titrate with 0.1 M cerric ammonium sulphate until yellow colour is produced. Perform a blank determination and make any necessary correction. Each ml of 0.1M cerric ammonium sulphate is equivalent to 0.00756 g of $C_8H_9NO_2$.

PROCEDURE

1. **For estimation of Paracetamol:**
   - **(a) Preparation of standard solution of Paracetamol (10 μg/ml)**
     - (i) Weigh accurately 100 mg of PCM powder and dissolve in 50 ml 0.1N HCl.
     - (ii) Make up the volume up to 100 ml by 0.1N HCl.
     - (iii) Take 10 ml of above solution and dilute to 100 ml with 0.1N HCl.
     - (iv) To get the resulting solution of 10 μg/ml concentration, take 10 ml and dilute to 100 ml with 0.1N HCl.
   - **(b) Preparation of sample solution of Paracetamol**
     - (i) Weigh and powder 20 tablets with the help of pestle mortar.
     - (ii) Weigh accurately a quantity of the powdered tablet equivalent to 0.100 gm of Paracetamol.
     - (iii) Extract the drug with three portions of 25–25 ml of 0.1N HCl.
     - (iv) Filter through Whatmann filter paper.
     - (v) Combine all the three filtrates and make up the volume up to 100 ml with 0.1N HCl.
     - (vi) Take 10 ml and dilute to 100 ml with 0.1N HCl.
     - (vii) To get the resulting solution, take 10 ml of above solution and dilute to 100 ml with 0.1N HCl.

     Measure the absorbance of both standard and sample at 244 nm and deduce the results by comparison.
2. **For estimation of Diclofenac sodium (DCLS)**
   - **(a) Preparation of standard solution of Diclofenac sodium (10 μg/ml)**
     - (i) Weigh accurately 100 mg of DCLS powder and dissolve in 50 ml 0.1N NaOH.
     - (ii) Make up the volume up to 100 ml by 0.1N NaOH.
     - (iii) Take 10 ml of above solution and dilute to 100 ml with 0.1N NaOH.
     - (iv) To get the resulting solution of 10 μg/ml concentration, take 10 ml and dilute to 100 ml with 0.1N NaOH.

(b) Preparation of sample solution of Diclofenac sodium

(i) The entire residue left after the extraction of Paracetamol as described above is used for the estimation of Diclofenac sodium.

(ii) Transfer the residue left on the filter paper to 100 ml volumetric flask with the help of 0.1N NaOH.

(iii) Make up the volumes up to 100 ml with 0.1N NaOH.

(iv) Take 10 ml of this solution of Diclofenac sodium and dilute to 100 ml with 0.1N NaOH.

(v) To get final concentration, take 10 ml of above solution and dilute to 100 ml with 0.1N NaOH.

Measure the absorbance of both the sample and standard solution at 276 nm and deduce the results by comparison.

OBSERVATIONS

1. Wt. variation test

S. No.	Wt. of tablets (gm)	S. No.	Wt. of tablets (gm)
1.	0.981	11.	0.980
2.	0.983	12.	0.974
3.	0.984	13.	0.986
4.	0.984	14.	0.975
5.	0.989	15.	0.985
6.	0.987	16.	0.971
7.	0.984	17.	0.989
8.	0.979	18.	0.978
9.	0.977	19.	0.976
10.	0.976	20.	0.982
	Average weight (gm)		0.980

2. Observed absorbance

S.No.	Drug	Absorbance	
		Standard	Test
1.	Paracetamol	0.708	0.615
2.	Diclofenac sodium	0.390	0.323

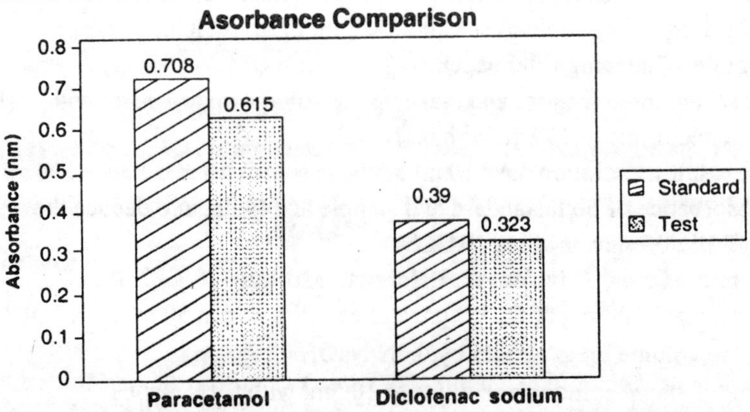

Label claim: Each tablet contains Paracetamol 0.325 gm and Diclofenac sodium 0.05 gm.

CALCULATION

1. Estimation of Paracetamol

$$C_2 = C_1 \times \frac{A_2}{A_1}$$

Where

A_1 = absorbance of standard Paracetamol solution = 0.708

A_2 = absorbance of test Paracetamol solution = 0.615

C_1 = concentration in gm/ml of standard Paracetamol solution

= 10×10^{-6} gm/ml

C_2 = concentration in gm/ml of test Paracetamol solution = ?

$$C_2 = 10 \times 10^{-6} \times \frac{0.615}{0.708}$$

$$= 8.6864 \times 10^{-6} \text{ gm/ml}$$

$$= \mathbf{8.6864\ \mu g/ml}$$

Calculation for % purity of Paracetamol sample

Theoretically the concentration of Paracetamol in test solution = 10 µg/ml.

Practically the concentration of Paracetamol in test solution is 8.6864 µg/ml.

$$\therefore \quad \% \text{ purity} = \frac{8.6864}{10} \times 100 = \mathbf{86.86\%\ w/w}$$

2. Estimation of Diclofenac sodium

$$C_2 = C_1 \times \frac{A_2}{A_1}$$

$$= 10 \times 10^{-6} \times \frac{0.323}{0.390}$$

$$= 8.282 \times 10^{-6} \text{ gm/ml}$$

i.e., **8.282 µg/ml.**

Calculation for % purity of Diclofenac sodium sample

Theoretically the concentration of Diclofenac sod. test solution = 10 µg/ml

Practically the concentration of Diclofenac solution in test solution = 8.282 µg/ml

$$\therefore \quad \% \text{ purity} = \frac{8.282}{10} \times 100$$

$$= \mathbf{82.82\%\ w/w}$$

RESULT

The percentage purity of Paracetamol and Diclofenac sodium in combination form by Spectrophotometric method was found to be 86.86% w/w and 82.82% w/w respectively.

EXPERIMENT 1.5B

Date ____________

ASSAY OF DICLOFENAC SODIUM AND PARACETAMOL
(Manual)

AIM

To carry out the analysis of diclofenac sodium and paracetamol in combined dosage form.

PROCEDURE

1. For estimation of Paracetamol:

(*a*) Preparation of standard solution of Paracetamol (10 μg/ml)

(*i*) Weigh accurately 100 mg of PCM powder and dissolve in 50 ml 0.1 N HCl.
(*ii*) Make up the volume up to 100 ml by 0.1 N HCl.
(*iii*) Take 10 ml of above solution and dilute to 100 ml with 0.1 N HCl.
(*iv*) To get the resulting solution of 10 μg/ml concentration, take 10 ml and dilute to 100 ml with 0.1N HCl.

(*b*) Preparation of sample solution of Paracetamol

(*i*) Weigh and powder 20 tablets with the help of pestle mortar.
(*ii*) Weigh accurately a quantity of the powdered tablet equivalent to 0.100 gm of Paracetamol.
(*iii*) Extract the drug with three portions of 25–25 ml of 0.1 N HCl.
(*iv*) Filter through Whatmann filter paper.
(*v*) Combine all the three filtrates and make up the volume up to 100 ml with 0.1 N HCl.
(*vi*) Take 10 ml and dilute to 100 ml with 0.1 N HCl.
(*vii*) To get the resulting solution, take 10 ml of above solution and dilute to 100 ml with 0.1 N HCl.

Measure the absorbance of both standard and sample at 244 nm and deduce the results by comparison.

2. For estimation of Diclofenac sodium (DCLS):

(*a*) Preparation of standard solution of Diclofenac sodium (10 μg/ml)

(*i*) Weigh accurately 100 mg of DCLS powder and dissolve in 50 ml 0.1 N NaOH.
(*ii*) Make up the volume up to 100 ml by 0.1 N NaOH.
(*iii*) Take 10 ml of above solution and dilute to 100 ml with 0.1 N NaOH.
(*iv*) To get the resulting solution of 10 μg/ml concentration, take 10 ml and dilute to 100 ml with 0.1 N NaOH.

(*b*) Preparation of sample solution of Diclofenac sodium

(*i*) The entire residue left after the extraction of Paracetamol as described above is used for the estimation of Diclofenac sodium.
(*ii*) Transfer the residue left on the filter paper to 100 ml volumetric flask with the help of 0.1N NaOH.
(*iii*) Make up the volume up to 100 ml with 0.1N NaOH.
(*iv*) Take 10 ml of this solution of Diclofenac sodium and dilute to 100 ml with 0.1N NaOH.
(*v*) To get final concentration, take 10 ml of above solution and dilute to 100 ml with 0.1N NaOH.

Measure the absorbance of both the sample and standard solution at 276 nm and deduce the results by comparison.

OBSERVATIONS

1. Wt. variation test

S. No.	Wt. of tablets (gm)	S. No.	Wt. of tablets (gm)
1.		11.	
2.		12.	
3.		13.	
4.		14.	
5.		15.	
6.		16.	
7.		17.	
8.		18.	
9.		19.	
10.		20.	
	Average weight (gm)		

2. Observed absorbance

S. No.	Drug	Absorbance	
		Standard	Test
1.	Paracetamol		
2.	Diclofenac sodium		

Absorbance Comparison

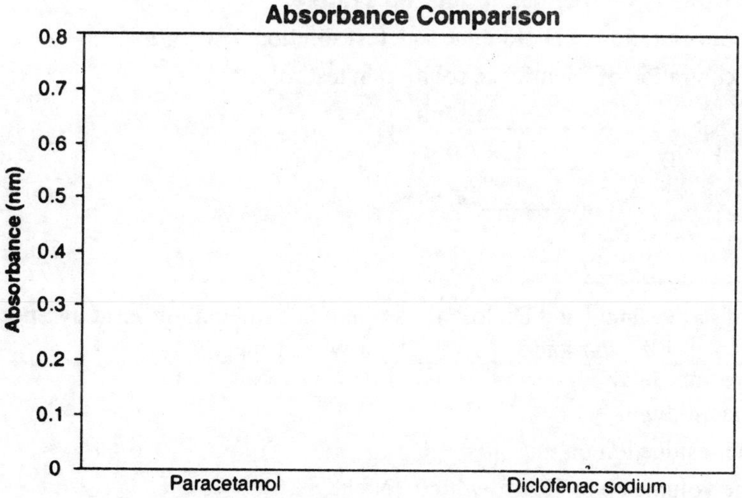

Label claim: Each tablet contains Paracetamol 0.325 gm and Diclofenac sodium 0.05 gm.

CALCULATION

1. Estimation of Paracetamol

$$C_2 = C_1 \times \frac{A_2}{A_1}$$

Where

A_1 = absorbance of standard Paracetamol solution = __________

A_2 = absorbance of test Paracetamol solution = __________

C_1 = concentration in gm/ml of standard Paracetamol solution

= __________ gm/ml

C_2 = concentration in gm/ml of test Paracetamol solution = ?

C_2 = ________ × ________

= ________

= ________

Calculation for % purity of Paracetamol sample:

Theoretically the concentration of Paracetamol in test solution = 10 µg/ml.

Practically the concentration of Paracetamol in test solution is ________ µg/ml.

= __________ % w/w

% Purity = __________ × 100

2. Estimation of Diclofenac solution

$$C_2 = C_1 \times \frac{A_2}{A_1}$$

C_2 = ________ × ________

= ________

= ________

i.e. __________ **µg/ml.**

Calculation for % purity of Diclofenac sodium sample:

Theoretically the concentration of Diclofenac sod. test solution = 10 µg/ml

Practically the concentration of Diclofenac solution in test solution

= __________ µg/ml

% Purity = ________ × 100

= __________ % w/w

RESULT

The percentage purity of Paracetamol and Diclofenac sodium in combination form by Spectrophotometric method was found to be __________ % w/w and __________ % w/w respectively.

EXPERIMENT 1.6A

Date ____________

EFFECT OF SOLVENTS ON λ_{max}

AIM

To study the effect of solvents upon the absorption spectrum of griseofulvin.

PRINCIPLE

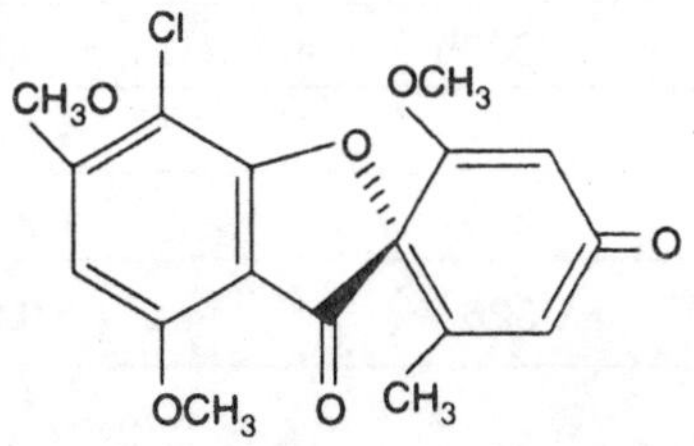

Solvent plays an important role in UV spectroscopy. The common solvents that used are water, methanol, ethanol, dilute acids, dilute alkalies etc. The solvents may cause salvation of the solute, ionic character, hydrogen bonding and salt effect, hence the solvent for a sample should be selected in such a manner that it should neither absorb in the region of absorption nor affect the absorption of the sample.

Mol. Formula: $C_{17}H_{17}ClO_6$ **Mol. Wt.:** 352.77

Griseofulvin is (2S, 4′R)-7-chloro-2′, 4, 6-trimethoxy-4′-methyl spiro [benzofuran-2(3H), 3′-cyclohexene]-3, 6′-diode produced by the growth of certain strains of Penicillium griseofulvin or obtained by any other means.

Category: Antifungal.

Solubility: Freely soluble in dimethylformamide and in 1, 1, 2, 2-tetrachloroethane soluble in acetone and in chloroform; slightly soluble in ethanol (95%) and in methanol; practically insoluble in water.

ASSAY

Weigh accurately about 80 mg and dissolve in sufficient ethanol to produce 200 ml. Dilute 2 ml to 100 ml with ethanol and measure the absorbance of the resulting solution at the maximum at about 291 nm as per I.P. 1996 (Appendix 5.5). Calculate the content of $C_{17}H_{17}ClO_6$ taking 686 as the value of A (1%, 1 cm) at the maximum at about 291 nm.

USES

Fungal infections of the skin, scalp, hair and nails where topical treatment has failed or is inappropriate.

PROCEDURE

1. Weigh accurately 100 mg of Griseofulvin powder and dissolve in 50 ml methanol (AR grade).
2. Make up the volume up to 100 ml by methanol.
3. Take 10 ml of above solution and dilute to 100 ml with methanol.
4. Get the resulting solution of 10 μg/ml concentration, take 10 ml and dilute to 100 ml with methanol.
5. In the same way, prepare the solution of Griseofulvin in 0.1 N NaOH, 0.1 N HCl and distilled water also.
6. Take any one of the solvent and observe the absorbance at different wavelengths against blank.
7. Take the dilution of the respective sample solution in the sample cell and find the absorbance and λ_{max} at different wavelengths.

8. Repeat the same procedure for the other solvents and sample solutions.
9. Plot a graph showing peaks and absorbance.
10. The peaks which shows maximum absorbance gives λ_{max}

OBSERVATIONS

(*a*) GSF in methanol (10 µg/ml)

S. No.	λ (nm)	Absorbance
1.	0	0
2.	236	0.413
3.	227	0.362
4.	293	0.470
5.	270	0.192
6.	325	0.083

(*b*) GSF in water (10 µg/ml)

S. No.	λ (nm)	Absorbance
1.	0	0
2.	296	0.485
3.	328	0.099
4.	330	0.102
5.	373	0.00
6.	372	0.219

(*c*) GSF in 0.1N HCl (10 µg/ml)

S. No.	λ (nm)	Absorbance
1.	0	0
2.	237	0.191
3.	246	0.162
4.	295	0.369
5.	375	– 0.1
6.	377	– 0.001

(*d*) GSF in 0.1N NaOH (10 µg/ml)

S. No.	λ (nm)	Absorbance
1.	0	0
2.	237	0.477
3.	383	0.001
4.	385	0.004

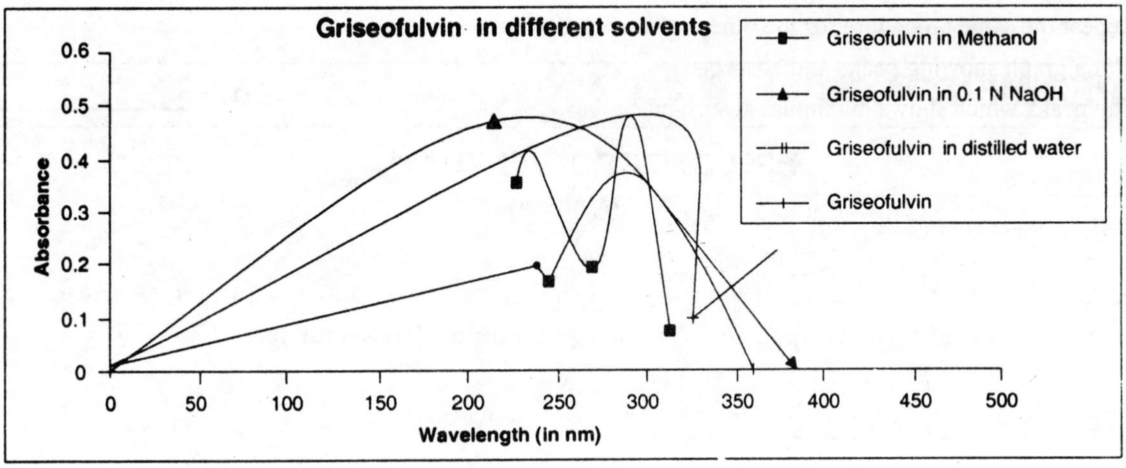

RESULTS

1. λ_{max} of GSF in methanol was found to be 293 nm.
2. λ_{max} of GSF in water was found to be 296 nm.
3. λ_{max} of GSF in 0.1N HCl was found to be 295 nm.
4. λ_{max} of GSF in 0.1N NaOH was found to be 237 nm.

EXPERIMENT 1.6B

Date ____________

EFFECT OF SOLVENTS ON λ_{max}
(Manual)

AIM

To study the effect of solvents upon the absorption spectrum of griseofulvin.

PROCEDURE

1. Weigh accurately 100 mg of Griseofulvin powder and dissolve in 50 ml methanol. (AR grade)
2. Make up the volume up to 100 ml by methanol.
3. Take 10 ml of above solution and dilute to 100 ml with methanol.
4. Get the resulting solution of 10 µg/ml concentration, take 10 ml and dilute to 100 ml with methanol.
5. In the same way, prepare the solution of Griseofulvin in 0.1N NaOH, 0.1N HCl and distilled water also.
6. Take any one of the solvent and observe the absorbance at different wavelengths against blank.
7. Take the dilution of the respective sample solution in the sample cell and find the absorbance and λ_{max} at different wavelengths.
8. Repeat the same procedure for the other solvents and sample solutions.
9. Plot a graph showing peaks and absorbance.
10. The peaks which shows maximum absorbance gives λ_{max}.

OBSERVATIONS

(*a*) GSF in methanol (10 µg/ml)

S. No.	λ (nm)	Absorbance
1.		
2.		
3.		
4.		
5.		
6.		
7.		

(*b*) GSF in water (10 µg/ml)

S. No.	λ (nm)	Absorbance
1.		
2.		
3.		
4.		
5.		
6.		

(*c*) **GSF in 0.1N HCl (10 μg/ml)**

S. No.	λ (nm)	Absorbance
1.		
2.		
3.		
4.		
5.		
6.		

(*d*) **GSF in 0.1N NaOH (10 μg/ml)**

S. No.	λ (nm)	Absorbance
1.		
2.		
3.		
4.		

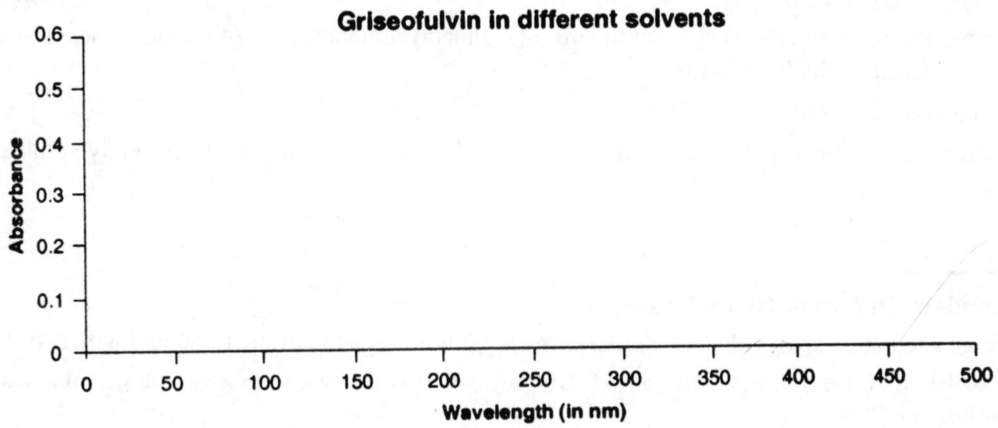

RESULTS

1. λ_{max} of GSF in methanol was found to be __________ nm.
2. λ_{max} of GSF in water was found to be __________ nm.
3. λ_{max} of GSF in 0.1N HCl was found to be __________ nm.
4. λ_{max} of GSF in 0.1N NaOH was found to be __________ nm.

EXPERIMENT 1.7 A

Date ______________

ASSAY OF DILTIAZEM HYDROCHLORIDE

AIM

To find out percentage purity of diltiazem HCl tablet IP by calibration curve method.

PRINCIPLE

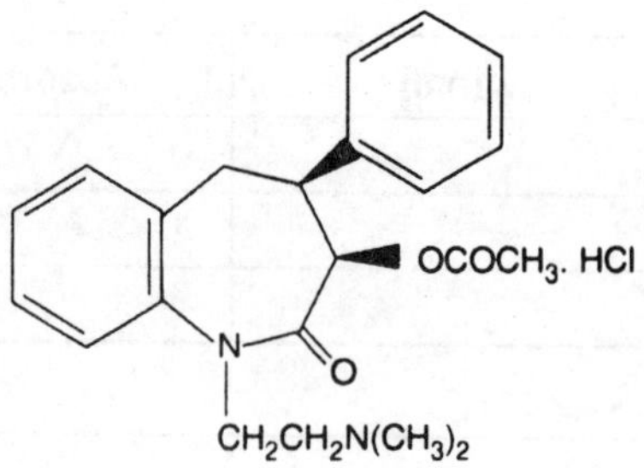

Mol. Formula: $C_{22}H_{26}N_2O_4S$. HCl **Mol. Wt.:** 450.98

Diltiazem hydrochloride is (+)-*cis*-2, 3, 4, 5-tetrahydro-5-(2-dimethylaminoethyl)-2-(4-methoxyphenyl)-4-oxobenzo[b] thiazepin-3-yl acetate monohydrochloride.

Category: Antianginal; calcium-channel blocker.

Solubility: Freely soluble in chloroform, in methanol, in water and in formic acid; sparingly soluble in ethanol; insoluble in ether.

PROCEDURE

A. For standard Diltiazem HCl solution

1. Weigh accurately about 100 mg of Diltiazem HCl (pure drug) and dilute to 100 ml with distilled water.
2. Take 10 ml of this solution and dilute to 100 ml with distilled water to give 100 μg/ml stock solution of Diltiazem HCl.
3. From the stock solution take 0.2 ml, 0.4 ml, 0.6 ml, 0.8 ml, 1.0 ml, 1.2 ml, 1.4 ml, 1.6 ml, 1.8 ml and 2.00 ml in different volumetric flasks of 10 ml each.
4. Dilute all the solutions to 10 ml with distilled water to give 2 μg/ml, 4 μg/ml, 6 μg/ml, 8 μg/ml, 10 μg/ml, 12 μg/ml, 14 μg/ml, 16 μg/ml, 18 μg/ml and 20 μg/ml respectively.
5. Run the samples into UV spectrophotometer for absorbance and plot the calibration curve by taking concentration on *X*-axis *vs.* absorbance on *Y*-axis at 247 nm.

B. For sample Diltiazem HCl dilution

1. Weigh accurately 20 tablets and calculate average weight of the tablets.
2. Powder the tablets with the help of mortar and pestle.
3. Weigh accurately powdered quantity of equivalent to 100 mg (0.1 gm) of Diltiazem HCl in volumetric flask.
4. To this powder, add 100 ml of methanol and dissolve using sonicator for 1 Hr.
5. Cool the solution at room temperature and centrifuge at 3500 rpm for 15 min.
6. Take 3.00 ml of this clear supernatant liquid and dilute to 10 ml with methanol.

7. From this solution, take 2 ml solution and further dilute to 100 ml with methanol, which gives the final concentration of 6 μg/ml.
8. Make sure that the resulting solution is clear and follows Beer's law.
9. Run the sample into UV spectrophotometer for absorbance at 247 nm.

OBSERVATIONS

1. Weight variation test

S. No.	Wt. of tablets (gm)	S. No.	Wt. of tablets (gm)
1.		11.	
2.		12.	
3.		13.	
4.		14.	
5.		15.	
6.		16.	
7.		17.	
8.		18.	
9.		19.	
10.		20.	
	Average weight (gm)		

2. Observations for standard dilutions of Diltiazem HCl

S. No.	Concentration (μg/ml)	Absorbance
1.	0.0	0.00
2.	2.00	0.135
3.	4.00	0.223
4.	6.00	0.325
5.	8.00	0.419
6.	10.00	0.514
7.	12.00	0.592
8.	14.00	0.698
9.	16.00	0.793
10.	18.00	0.872
11.	20.00	0.980
12.	Sample	**0.313**

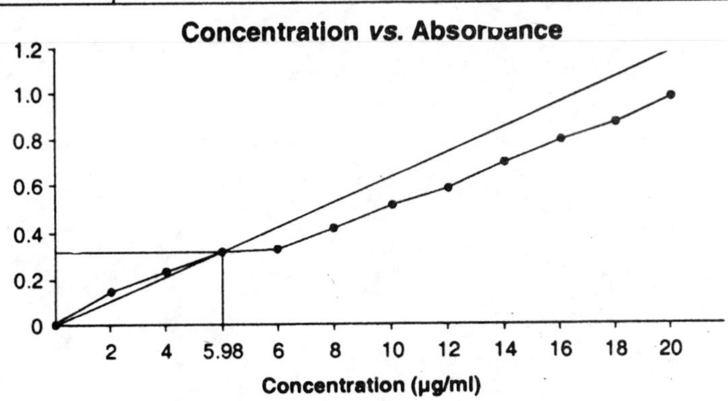

The absorbance for test solution (sample) = 0.313

Theoretical concentration of sample solution:

100 mg of DZM HCl diluted to 100 ml with methanol = 1 mg/ml.

When 3 ml of 1 mg/ml concentration diluted to 10 ml with methanol = 300 μg/ml.

2 ml of 300 μg/ml concentration diluted to 100 ml with methanol = 6 μg/ml.

So final concentration = 6 μg/ml.

CALCULATIONS

$$y = mx + c$$

Where

x = concentration of sample solution

m = 0.0476

y = absorption of sample solution

c = 0.0284 (from graph)

$$\therefore \quad 0.313 = 0.0476x + 0.0284$$

$$\therefore \quad x = \frac{0.313 - 0.0284}{0.0476}$$

$$= \mathbf{5.98\ \mu g/ml}$$

Concentration of sample solution as per label claim (Theoretically)

$$= 6\ \mu g/ml$$

$$\therefore \quad \%\ \text{purity} = \frac{\text{Practically found concentration}}{\text{Theoretical concentration}} \times 100$$

$$= \frac{5.98}{6.00} \times 100$$

$$= \mathbf{99.6\%\ w/w}$$

RESULT

The % purity of given sample of Diltiazem HCl tablet by Spectrophotometry using calibration curve method was found to be **99.6% w/w.**

EXPERIMENT 1.7B

Date ____________

ASSAY OF DILTIAZEM HYDROCHLORIDE
(Manual)

AIM

To find out percentage purity of diltiazem HCl tablet IP by calibration curve method.

PROCEDURE

A. For standard Diltiazem HCl solution

1. Weigh accurately about 100 mg of Diltiazem HCl (pure drug) and dilute to 100 ml with distilled water.
2. Take 10 ml of this solution and dilute to 100 ml with distilled water to give 100 μg/ml stock solution of Diltiazem HCl.
3. From the stock solution take 0.2 ml, 0.4 ml, 0.6 ml, 0.8 ml, 1.0 ml, 1.2 ml, 1.4 ml, 1.6 ml, 1.8 ml and 2.00 ml in different volumetric flasks of 10 ml each.
4. Dilute all the solutions to 10 ml with distilled water to give 2 μg/ml, 4 μg/ml, 6 μg/ml, 8 μg/ml, 10 μg/ml, 12 μg/ml, 14 μg/ml, 16 μg/ml, 18 μg/ml and 20 μg/ml respectively.
5. Run the samples into UV spectrophotometer for absorbance and plot the calibration curve by taking concentration on *X*-axis *vs.* absorbance on *Y*-axis at 247 nm.

B. For sample Diltiazem HCl dilution

1. Weigh accurately 20 tablets and calculate average weight of the tablets.
2. Powder the tablets with the help of mortar and pestle.
3. Weigh accurately powdered quantity of equivalent to 100 mg (0.1 gm) of Diltiazem HCl in volumetric flask.
4. To this powder, add 100 ml of methanol and dissolve using sonicator for 1 Hr.
5. Cool the solution at room temperature and centrifuge at 3500 rpm for 15 min.
6. Take 3.00 ml of this clear supernatant liquid and dilute to 10 ml with methanol.
7. From this solution, take 2 ml solution and further dilute to 100 ml with methanol which gives the final concentration of 6 μg/ml.
8. Make sure that the resulting solution is clear and follows Beer's law.
9. Run the sample into UV spectrophotometer for absorbance at 247 nm.

OBSERVATIONS

1. Weight variation test

S. No.	Wt. of tablets (gm)	S. No.	Wt. of tablets (gm)
1.		11.	
2.		12.	
3.		13.	
4.		14.	
5.		15.	
6.		16.	
7.		17.	
8.		18.	
9.		19.	
10.		20.	
	Average weight (gm)		

2. Observations for standard dilutions of Diltiazem HCl

S. No.	Concentration (μg/ml)	Absorbance
1.	0.0	
2.	2.0	
3.	4.0	
4.	6.0	
5.	8.0	
6.	10.0	
7.	12.0	
8.	14.0	
9.	16.0	
10.	18.0	
11.	20.0	
12.	Sample	

Concentration *vs.* Absorbance

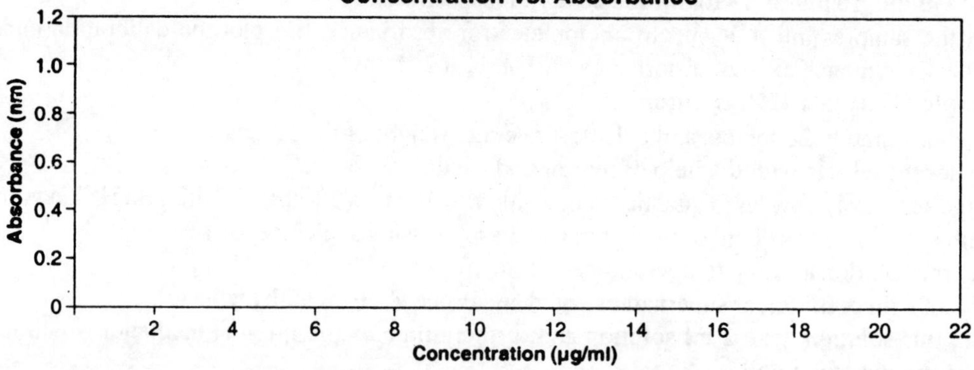

The absorbance for test solution (Sample) = __________

Theoretical concentration of sample solution:

100 mg of DZM HCl diluted to 100 ml with methanol = 1 mg/ml.

When 3 ml of 1 mg/ml concentration diluted to 10 ml with methanol = ________μg/ml.

2 ml of 300 μg/ml concentration diluted to 100 ml with methanol =__________μg/ml.

So final concentration =__________μg/ml.

CALCULATIONS

$y = mx + c$

Where x = concentration of sample solution

m = __________

y = absorption of sample solution

c = ________ (from graph)

________ = ________ x + ________

$$x = \frac{\_\_\_\_\_\_ - \_\_\_\_\_\_}{\_\_\_\_\_\_}$$

$\therefore \quad x$ ______ = __________ **µg/ml**

Concentration of sample solution as per label claim (Theoretically)

= _________ µg/ml

$$\therefore \quad \%\ \text{purity} = \frac{\text{Practically found concentration}}{\text{Theoretical concentration}} \times 100$$

= _________ × 100

= __________ **% w/w**

RESULT

The % purity of given sample of Diltiazem HCl tablet by Spectrophotometry using calibration curve method was found to be__________ **% w/w.**

EXPERIMENT 1.8A

Date ____________

STUDY OF λ_{max} OF DILTIAZEM HCl IN DIFFERENT SOLVENTS

AIM

To find out λ_{max} of diltiazem HCl in different solvents.

PRINCIPLE

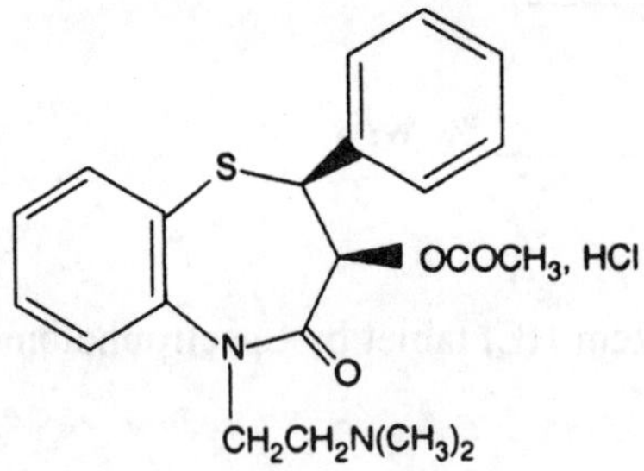

Mol. Formula: $C_{22}H_{26}N_2O_4S$, HCl **Mol. Wt.:** 450.98

Diltiazem hydrochloride is (+)-*cis*-2, 3, 4, 5-tetrahydro-5-(2-dimethylaminoethyl)-2-(4-methoxyphenyl)-4-oxobenzo[b] thiazepin-3-yl acetate monohydrochloride.

Category: Antianginal; calcium-channel blocker.

Description: White crystalline powder or small crystals.

Solubility: Freely soluble in chloroform, in methanol, in water and in formic acid; sparingly soluble in ethanol; insoluble in ether.

PROCEDURE

1. Weigh accurately about 100 mg of DZM HCl and dissolve in 100 ml of distilled water.
2. Take 10 ml of this solution and dilute to 100 ml with distilled water and label as stock solution.
3. Take 0.5 ml of this stock solution in four different volumetric flasks each of 10 ml.
4. Make up the volume up to 10 ml with Methanol, 0.1N NaOH, 0.1N HCl and distilled water to get 5 µg/ml of Diltiazem HCl concentration.
5. Determine the λ_{max} of 5 µg/ml concentration samples at different wavelengths.

OBSERVATIONS

Diltiazem HCl in different solvents (5 µg/ml):

Methanol		0.1N NaOH		Distilled water		0.1N HCl	
Abs.	λ	Abs.	λ	Abs.	λ	Abs.	λ
0	0	0	0	0	229	0	0
238	0.37	0.475	238	0.459	235	0.326	238
223	0.243	0.007	349	0	328	– 0.06	299
		0.008	371	0.002	347	– 0.01	359
		0.001	377	0	358	– 0.02	377
		0.007	379				
		0.001	383				
		0.001	391				

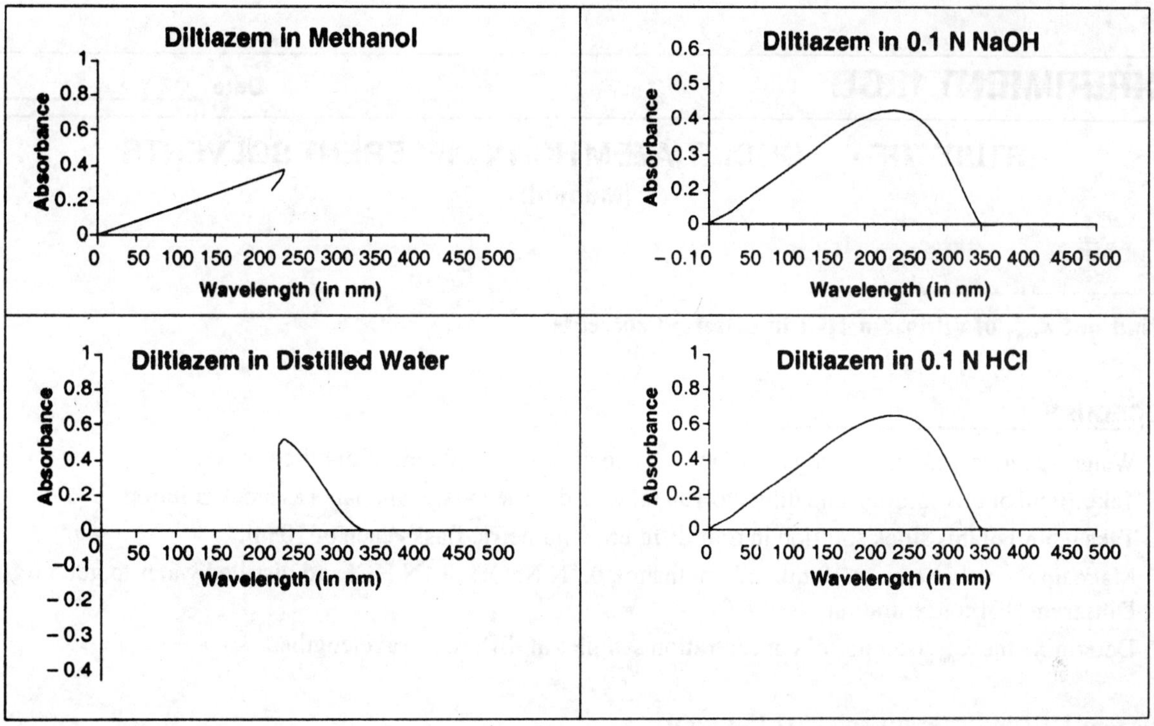

RESULT

1. λ_{max} of Diltiazem HCl in methanol was found to be 238 nm.
2. λ_{max} of Diltiazem HCl in 0.1N NaOH was found to be 238 nm.
3. λ_{max} of Diltiazem HCl in distilled water was found to be 235 nm.
4. λ_{max} of Diltiazem HCl in 0.1 N HCl was found to be 238 nm.

EXPERIMENT 1.8B

Date ____________

STUDY OF λ_{max} OF DILTIAZEM HCl IN DIFFERENT SOLVENTS
(Manual)

AIM

To find out λ_{max} of diltiazem HCl in different solvents.

PROCEDURE

1. Weigh accurately about 100 mg of DZM HCl and dissolve in 100 ml of distilled water.
2. Take 10 ml of this solution and dilute to 100 ml with distilled water and label as stock solution.
3. Take 0.5 ml of this stock solution in four different volumetric flasks each of 10 ml.
4. Make up the volume up to 10 ml with methanol, 0.1N NaOH, 0.1N HCl and distilled water to get 5 μg/ml of Diltiazem HCl concentration.
5. Determine the λ_{max} of 5 μg/ml concentration samples at different wavelengths.

Diltiazem HCl in different solvents (5 μg/ml):

Methanol		0.1N NaOH		Distilled water		0.1N HCl	
Abs.	λ	Abs.	λ	Abs.	λ	Abs.	λ

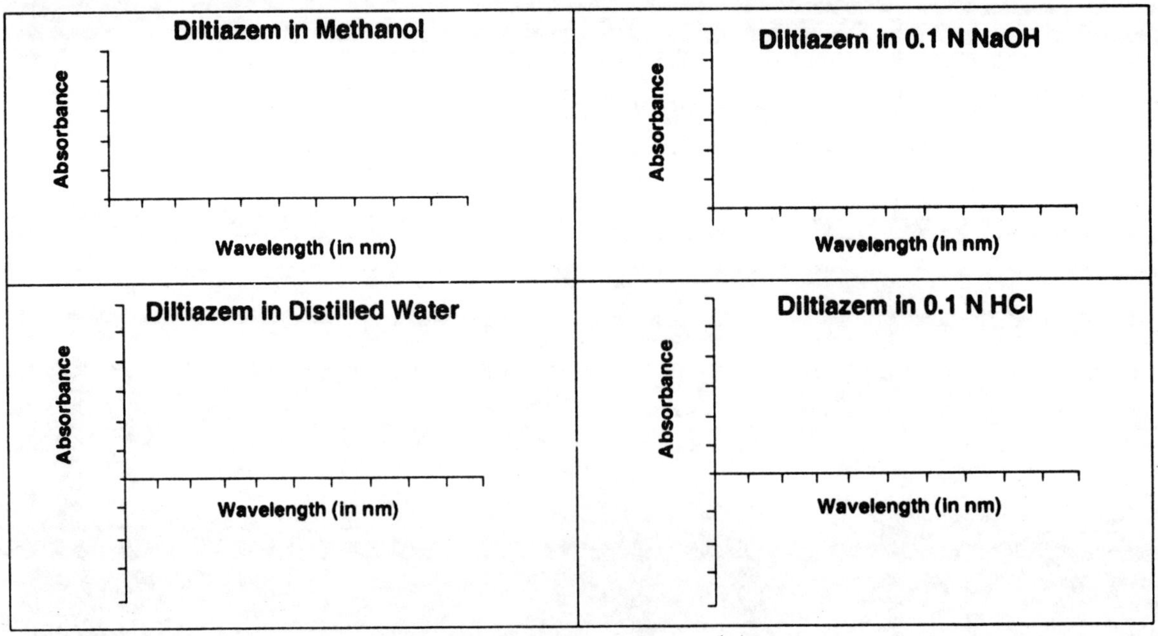

RESULTS

1. λ_{max} of Diltiazem HCl in methanol was found to be __________ nm.
2. λ_{max} of Diltiazem HCl in 0.1N NaOH was found to be __________ nm.
3. λ_{max} of Diltiazem HCl in distilled water was found to be __________ nm.
4. λ_{max} of Diltiazem HCl in 0.1 N HCl was found to be __________ nm.

EXPERIMENT 1.9 A

Date ____________

ASSAY OF CHLORAMPHENICOL CAPSULES I.P.

AIM

To determine percentage purity of the given sample of chloramphenicol capsules I.P.

PRINCIPLE

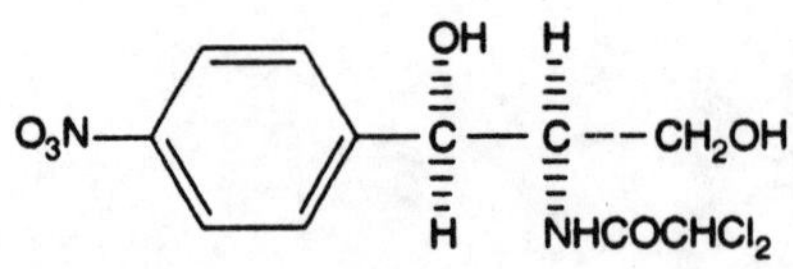

Mol. Formula: $C_{11}H_{12}Cl_2N_2O_5$ **Mol. Wt.:** 323.13

Chloramphenicol is 2, 2-dichloro-*N*-[(α-*R*, β-*R*)-β *55D*-hydroxy-α-hydroxymethyl-4-nitrophenethyl] acetamide. It is produced by the growth of certain strains of Streptomyces venezuelae in a suitable medium, but is normally prepared by synthesis.

Category: Antibacterial.

Description: White to grayish-white or yellowish-white, fine crystalline powder or fine-crystals, needles or elongated plates; odourless.

Solubility: Freely soluble in ethanol (95%) and in 1, 2-propanediol; slightly soluble in water and in ether.

ASSAY

Weigh accurately about 0.125 g and dissolve in sufficient water to produce 250 ml. Dilute 10 ml with sufficient water to produce 250 ml. Measure the absorbance of the resulting solution at the maximum at abcut 278 nm. Calculate the content of $C_{11}H_{12}Cl_2N_2O_5$ taking 297 as the value A (1%, 1 cm) at the maximum at about 278 nm.

USES

Severe life-threatening infections, particularly those caused by Haemophilus influenzae, and typhoid fever; also, cerebral abscess; mastoiditis; relapsing fever; gangrene; granuloma inguinale; listeriosis; severe melioidosis; plague; psitticosis; tularaemia; Whipple disease; septicaemia; empirical treatment of meningitis.

PROCEDURE

1. Weigh 20 capsules and mix the contents.
2. Weigh accurately a quantity of powdered drug equivalent to 0.200 gm of Chloramphenicol.
3. Dissolve in 800 ml with distilled water, warm gently (if necessary) to get a clear solution.
4. Dilute to 1000 ml with distilled water.
5. Take 10 ml of above solution and dilute to 100 ml in order to get the resulting solution.
6. Measure the absorbance at 278 nm $\left(E^{1\%}_{1cm}\ 298\right)$.

OBSERVATION

1. Weight variation

S. No.	Wt. of capsule (gm)	Wt. of content of capsule (gm)	Average wt. of content of capsule
1.	0.632	0.608	
2.	0.643	0.600	
3.	0.678	0.592	
4.	0.643	0.610	
5.	0.623	0.590	
6.	0.654	0.606	
7.	0.632	0.600	
8.	0.656	0.597	
9.	0.698	0.601	
10.	0.656	0.600	
11.	0.623	0.599	$\frac{11.6}{20} = 0.580$ gm
12.	0.624	0.612	
13.	0.621	0.588	
14.	0.631	0.607	
15.	0.632	0.600	
16.	0.633	0.593	
17.	0.631	0.581	
18.	0.635	0.606	
19.	0.626	0.594	
20.	0.627	0.619	

Avg. wt. of content of one capsule = 0.580 gm

Label claimed = 0.500 gm

2. Absorbance = 0.595

CALCULATION

$\because$ 0.580 gm of powder content = 0.500 gm of Chloramphenicol

$\therefore$ x gm of powder content = 0.200 gm of Chloramphenicol

$$\therefore \quad x = \frac{0.200 \times 0.580}{0.500} = 0.232 \text{ gm}$$

So 0.232 gm of powder content $\equiv$ 0.200 gm of Chloramphenicol

DILUTION FACTOR

$$\text{Dilution Factor} = \frac{0.232}{1000} \times \frac{10}{100} \times 100$$

$$= 0.00232\%\ \text{w/v}$$

FORMULA

$$\%\ \text{Purity} = \frac{A}{E} \times \frac{\text{Avg. wt.}}{\text{L.C.}} \times \frac{100}{\text{D.F.}}$$

$$= \frac{0.595}{298} \times \frac{0.580}{0.500} \times \frac{100}{0.00232}$$

$$= 99.83\%$$

RESULT

The percentage purity of the given sample of Chloramphenicol capsule was found to be 99.83% w/w.

EXPERIMENT 1.9B

Date ______________

ASSAY OF CHLORAMPHENICOL CAPSULE I.P.

(Manual)

AIM

To determine percentage purity of the given sample of chloramphenicol capsules I.P. by spectrophotometric method.

PROCEDURE

1. Weigh 20 capsules and mix the contents.
2. Weigh accurately a quantity of powdered drug equivalent to 0.200 gm of Chloramphenicol.
3. Dissolve in 800 ml with distilled water, warm gently (if necessary) to get a clear solution.
4. Dilute to 1000 ml with distilled water.
5. Take 10 ml of above solution and dilute to 100 ml in order to get the resulting solution.
6. Measure the absorbance at 278 nm $\left(E_{1cm}^{1\%}\ 298\right)$.

OBSERVATION

1. Weight variation

S. No.	Wt. of capsule (gm)	Wt. of content of capsule (gm)	Average wt. of content of capsule
1.			
2.			
3.			
4.			
5.			
6.			
7.			
8.			
9.			
10.			
11.			
12.			
13.			
14.			
15.			
16.			
17.			
18.			
19.			
20.			

Avg. wt. of content of one capsule = ________ gm

Label claimed = 0.500 gm

2. Absorbance = ________

CALCULATION

∵ gm of powder content = 0.500 gm of Chloramphenicol

∴ x gm of powder content = ________ gm of Chloramphenicol

$$x = \frac{\_\_\_\_\_ \times \_\_\_\_\_}{\_\_\_\_\_}$$

= ________ gm

So ________ gm of powder content ≡ 0.200 gm of Chloramphenicol.

DILUTION FACTOR

Dilution factor = ________ × ________ × 100

= ________ % w/v

FORMULA

$$\% \text{ Purity} = \frac{A}{E} \times \frac{\text{Avg. wt.}}{\text{L.C.}} \times \frac{100}{\text{D.F.}}$$

= ________ × ________ × 100

= ________%

RESULT

The % purity of the given sample of Chloramphenicol capsule was found to be ________% w/w.

EXPERIMENT 1.10 A

Date ____________

ASSAY OF FUROSEMIDE INJECTION I.P.

AIM

To determine the percentage purity of given sample of furosemide injection I.P.

PRINCIPLE

FUROSEMIDE (FRUSEMIDE)

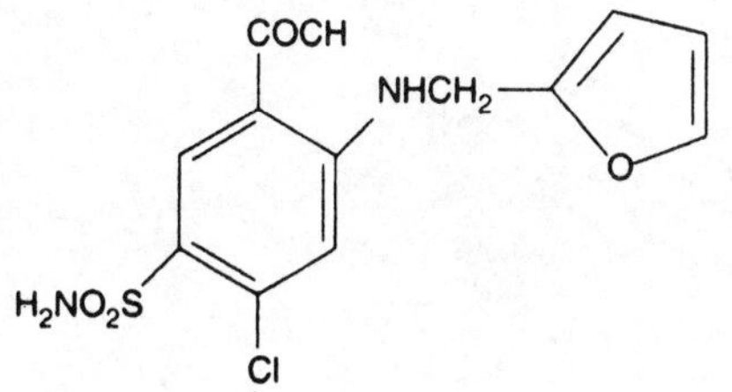

Mol. Formula: $C_{12}H_{11}ClN_2O_5S$ **Mol. Wt.:** 330.74

Furosemide is 4-chloro-N-furfuryl-5-sulphamoylanthranilic acid.

Category: Diuretic.

Description: White or almost white, crystalline powder.

Solubility: Soluble in acetone; sparingly soluble in ethanol (95%); slightly soluble in ether; practically insoluble in water. It dissolves in dilute aqueous solutions of alkali hydroxides.

ASSAY

1. Weigh accurately about 0.5 g, dissolve in 40 ml of dimethylformamide and titrate with 0.1M sodium hydroxide using bromothymol blue solution as indicator. Perform a blank determination and make any necessary correction.

   Each ml of 0.1M sodium hydroxide is equivalent to 0.03307 g of $C_{12}H_{11}ClN_2O_5S$.

2. Weigh and powder 20 tablets. Weigh accurately a quantity of the powder equivalent to about 0.1 g of Furosemide and shake with 150 ml of 0.1M sodium hydroxide for 10 minutes. Add sufficient 0.1M Sodium hydroxide to produce 250 ml and filter. Dilute 5.0 ml to 200 ml with 0.1 M sodium hydroxide and measure the absorbance of the resulting solution at the maximum at about 271 nm. Calculate the content of $C_{12}H_{11}ClN_2O_5S$ taking 580 as the value of A(1%, 1 cm) at the maximum at about 271 nm.

USES

An example of a loop diuretic.

PROCEDURE

1. Measure the exact 2 ml volume equivalent to about 20 mg of Furosemide injection.
2. Dilute to 100 ml with distilled water.
3. Take 5 ml of the above solution and dilute to 100 ml with 0.1N NaOH solution.
4. Measure the absorbance of the resulting solution at 271 nm against blank solution.

OBSERVATION

1. Label claim

   Each ml of Furosemide injection contains

   $$= 10 \text{ mg of Furosemide} = 0.01 \text{ gm}$$

   $$\text{So for 20 mg of Furosemide} = \frac{0.02}{0.01} = 2 \text{ ml}$$

2. $$\text{Observed absorbance (A)} = 0.556$$

3. $$\text{Dilution Factor} = \frac{0.02}{100} \times \frac{5}{100} \times 100$$

   $$= 0.001 \text{ gm\% w/v}$$

4. $$\text{\% purity} = \frac{A}{E_{1\text{cm}}^{1\%}} \times \frac{100}{\text{D.F.}}$$

   $$= \frac{0.569}{580} \times \frac{1}{0.001} \times \frac{100}{1}$$

   $$= 98.10\%$$

RESULT

The percentage purity of given sample of Furosemide injection I.P. was found to be 98.10% w/v.

EXPERIMENT 1.10B

Date ____________

ASSAY OF FUROSEMIDE INJECTION I.P.

(Manual)

AIM

To determine the percentage purity of given sample of furosemide injection I.P.

PROCEDURE

1. Measure the exact 2 ml volume equivalent to about 20 mg of Furosemide injection.
2. Dilute to 100 ml with distilled water.
3. Take 5 ml of the above solution and dilute to 100 ml with 0.1N NaOH solution.
4. Measure the absorbance of the resulting solution at 271 nm against blank solution.

OBSERVATION

1. Label claim

   Each ml of Furosemide injection contains

   = 10 mg of Furosemide = __________ gm

   So for 20 mg of Furosemide = __________ ml

2. Observed absorbance (A) = __________

   = __________ × __________ × 100

3. Dilution Factor = ____________ gm% w/v

4. % purity $= \dfrac{A}{E^{1\%}_{1cm}} \times \dfrac{100}{D.F.}$

   = __________ × __________ × __________

   = __________ %

RESULT

The percentage purity of given sample of Furosemide injection I.P. was found to be __________ % w/v.

EXPERIMENT 1.11A

Date ____________

ASSAY OF ALLOPURINOL

AIM

To determine the percentage purity of given sample of allopurinol tablets I.P.

PRINCIPLE

ALLOPURINOL

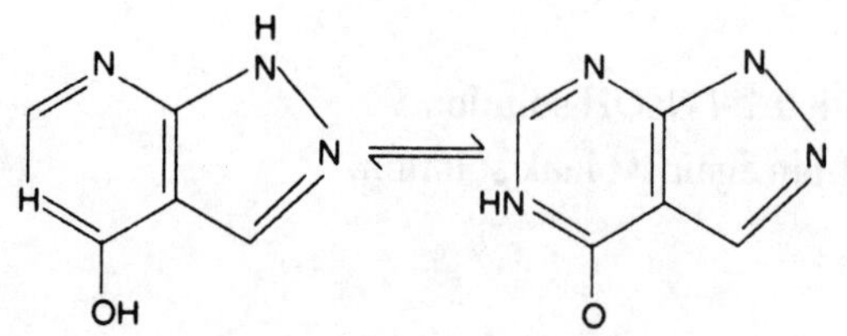

Mol. Formula: $C_5H_4N_4O$ **Mol. Wt.:** 136.11

Allopurinol is a tautomeric mixture of 1*H*-pyrazolo [3,4-*d*]- pyrimidin-4-ol and 1,5-dihydro-4*H*-pyrazolo [3,4-*d*]-pyrimidin-4-one.

Category: Gout therapy.

Description: White or almost white, crystalline powder.

Solubility: Very slightly soluble in water and in ethanol (95%); practically insoluble in chloroform and in ether. It is soluble in dilute solutions of alkali hydroxides.

ASSAY

Weigh accurately about 0.2 g, dissolve with gentle heating, if necessary, in 50 ml of dimethylformamide and carry out the method A for non-aqueous titration given in I.P. 1996 (Appendix 3.45) using 0.1M tetrabutylammonium hydroxide as the titrant and determining the end-point potentiometrically. Each ml of 0.1M tetrabutylammonium hydroxide is equivalent to 0.01361 g of $C_5H_4N_4O$.

USES

Prophylaxis of gout and hyperuricaemia.

PROCEDURE

1. Weigh and powder 20 tablets with the help of mortar and pestle.
2. Weigh accurately a quantity of the powdered tablets equivalent to 0.100 gm of Allopurinol.
3. Add 10 ml of 0.1M NaOH and dilute 100 ml with 0.1M HCl.
4. Take 10 ml of the solution and dilute to 100 ml with 0.1M HCl.
5. Take 10 ml of resulting solution and again dilute to 100 ml with 0.1M HCl.
6. Measure the absorbance at 250 nm.

OBSERVATION

1. Weight variation test

S. No.	Wt. of tablets (gm)	S. No.	Wt. of tablets (gm)	Avg. wt. (gm)
1.	0.175	11.	0.178	$\frac{3.49}{20} = 0.1745$ gm
2.	0.175	12.	0.170	
3.	0.177	13.	0.175	
4.	0.174	14.	0.174	
5.	0.172	15.	0.177	
6.	0.174	16.	0.172	
7.	0.170	17.	0.174	
8.	0.174	18.	0.174	
9.	0.178	19.	0.175	
10.	0.174	20.	0.174	

2. Observed absorbance (A) = 0.578

CALCULATION

1. Label claim of given tablet = 0.100 gm
2. Wt. of 20 tablets = 3.49 gm
3. Average wt. of 1 tablet = 0.1745 gm

∵ 0.1745 gm of powder = 0.100 gm of Allopurinol

∴ 0.100 gm of Allopurinol = 0.1745 gm of powder drug.

$$\text{D.F.} = \frac{0.1745}{100} \times \frac{10}{100} \times \frac{10}{100} \times 100$$

$$= 0.001745 \text{ gm \% w/v}$$

FORMULA

$$\% \text{ purity} = \frac{A}{E^{1\%}_{1\text{cm}}} \times \frac{\text{Avg. wt.}}{\text{L.C.}} \times \frac{100}{\text{D.F.}}$$

$$= \frac{0.578}{563} \times \frac{0.1745}{0.100} \times \frac{100}{0.001745}$$

$$= 102.66\%$$

RESULT

The % purity of given sample of 0.100 gm of Allopurinol tablet I.P. was found to be 102.66% w/w.

EXPERIMENT 1.11 B

Date ________

ASSAY OF ALLOPURINOL
(Manual)

AIM

To determine the percentage purity of given sample of allopurinol tablets I.P.

PRINCIPLE

$$E^{1\%}_{1\,cm} = 563, \lambda_{max} = 250 \text{ nm}$$

PROCEDURE

1. Weigh and powder 20 tablets with the help of mortar and pestle.
2. Weigh accurately a quantity of the powdered tablets equivalent to 0.100 gm of Allopurinol.
3. Add 10 ml of 0.1M NaOH and dilute 100 ml with 0.1M HCl.
4. Take 10 ml of the solution and dilute to 100 ml with 0.1M HCl.
5. Take 10 ml of resulting solution and again dilute to 100 ml with 0.1M HCl.
6. Measure the absorbance at 250 nm.

OBSERVATION

1. Weight variation test

S. No.	Wt. of tablets (gm)	S. No.	Wt. of tablets (gm)	Avg. wt. (gm)
1.		11.		
2.		12.		
3.		13.		
4.		14.		
5.		15.		
6.		16.		
7.		17.		
8.		18.		
9.		19.		
10.		20.		

2. Observed absorbance (A) = ________

CALCULATION

1. Label claim of given tablet = 0.100 gm
2. Wt. of 20 tablets = ________ gm
3. Average wt. of 1 tablet = ________ gm

∵ ________ gm of powder = 0.100 gm of Allopurinol

∴ 0.100 gm of Allopurinol = ________ gm of powder drug.

= ________ × ________ × ________ × 100

D.F. = ________ gm % w/v

FORMULA

$$\% \text{ purity} = \frac{A}{E^{1\%}_{1\text{ cm}}} \times \frac{\text{Avg. wt}}{\text{L.C.}} \times \frac{100}{\text{D.F.}}$$

= ________ × ________ × ________

= ________%

RESULT

The percentage purity of given sample of 0.100 gm of Allopurinol tablet I.P. was found to be ________% w/w.

EXPERIMENT 1.12A

Date ____________

ASSAY OF PROPRANOLOL HCl TABLETS I.P.

AIM

To determine the percentage purity of given sample of propranolol HCl tablets.

PRINCIPLE

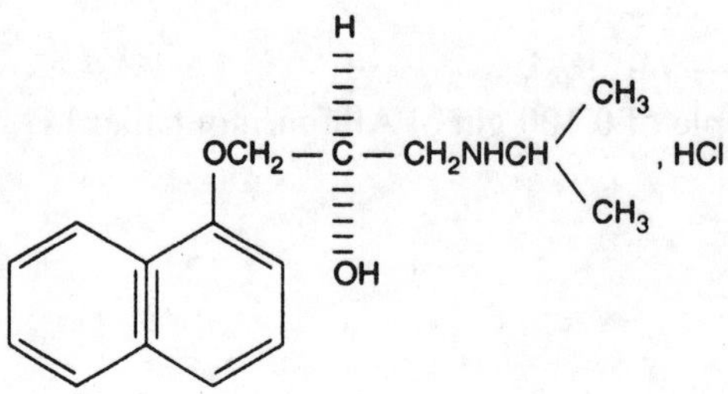

Mol. Formula: $C_{16}H_{21}NO_2$, HCl **Mol. Wt.:** 295.81

Propranolol hydrochloride is (*RS*)-1-isopropylamino-3-(1-naphthyloxy) propan-2-ol hydrochloride.

Category: Beta-adrenoceptor antagonist (antihypertensive, antianginal and antiarrhythmic agent).

Description: White or almost white powder.

Solubility: Soluble in water and in ethanol (95%); slightly soluble in chloroform; practically insoluble in ether.

USES

Prophylaxis of migraine

$$E^{1\%}_{1\,cm} = 222$$

PROCEDURE

1. Weigh and powder 20 tablets.
2. Weigh accurately a quantity of powdered tablets equivalent to 0.020 gm of Propranolol HCl.
3. Shake with 20 ml of distilled water for 10 minutes.
4. To this solution, add 50 ml of methanol and again shake for further 10 minutes.
5. Dilute to 100 ml, the above solution with methanol and filter in order to get a clear solution.
6. Take 10 ml of the filtrate and dilute to 50 ml with methanol.
7. Measure the absorbance of the resulting solution at 290 nm.

OBSERVATIONS

1. Weight variation test

S. No.	Wt. of tablets (gm)	Avg. wt. (gm)
1.	0.200	
2.	0.202	
3.	0.209	
4.	0.193	
5.	0.196	
6.	0.206	
7.	0.200	
8.	0.202	
9.	0.204	
10.	0.198	$\frac{402}{20} = 0.201$ gm
11.	0.201	
12.	0.200	
13.	0.201	
14.	0.202	
15.	0.201	
16.	0.202	
17.	0.204	
18.	0.196	
19.	0.206	
20.	0.205	

2. Observed absorbance (A) = 0.586

CALCULATIONS

1. Label claim of given tablet = 0.04 gm
2. Wt. of 20 tablets = 4.02 gm
3. Avg. wt. of 1 tablet = 0.201 gm

0.201 gm of powder = 0.04 gm of Propranolol HCl

∴ x gm of powder ≡ 0.02 gm of Propranolol HCl

$$\therefore \quad x = \frac{0.02 \times 0.201}{0.04} \Rightarrow 0.1005 \text{ gm}$$

$$\% \text{ D.F.} = \frac{0.1005}{100} \times \frac{10}{50} \times 100 = 0.0201\% \text{ w/v}$$

$$\% \text{ purity} = \frac{A}{E_{1\text{cm}}^{1\%}} \times \frac{\text{Avg. wt.}}{\text{L.C.}} \times \frac{100}{\text{D.F.}}$$

$$= \frac{0.586}{222} \times \frac{0.201}{0.04} \times \frac{100}{0.0201}$$

$$= 65.99\%$$

RESULT

The percentage purity of given sample of 0.04 gm of Propranolol HCl tablet I.P. was found to be 65.99%.

EXPERIMENT 1.12B

Date ____________

ASSAY OF PROPRANOLOL HCl TABLETS I.P.
(Manual)

AIM

To determine the percentage purity of given sample of propranolol HCl tablets.

PRINCIPLE

$$E^{1\%}_{1cm} = 222$$

PROCEDURE

1. Weigh and powder 20 tablets.
2. Weigh accurately a quantity of powdered tablets equivalent to 0.020 gm of Propranolol HCl.
3. Shake with 20 ml of distilled water for 10 minutes.
4. To this solution, add 50 ml of methanol and again shake for further 10 minutes.
5. Dilute to 100 ml, the above solution with methanol and filter in order to get a clear solution.
6. Take 10 ml of the filtrate and dilute to 50 ml with methanol.
7. Measure the absorbance of the resulting solution at 290 nm.

OBSERVATIONS

1. Weight variation test

S. No.	Wt. of tablets (gm)	Avg. wt. (gm)
1.		
2.		
3.		
4.		
5.		
6.		
7.		
8.		
9.		
10.		
11.		
12.		
13.		
14.		

(Contd.)

S. No.	Wt. of tablets (gm)	Avg. wt. (gm)
15.		
16.		
17.		
18.		
19.		
20.		

2. Observed absorbance (A) = __________

CALCULATIONS

1. Label claim of given tablet = 0.04 gm
2. Wt. of 20 tablets = __________ gm
3. Avg. wt. of 1 tablet = __________ gm

__________ gm of powder = 0.04 gm of Propranolol HCl

∴ *x* gm of powder = __________ gm of Propranolol HCl

$$x = \frac{\_\_\_\_ \times \_\_\_\_}{\_\_\_\_}$$

= __________ gm

% D.F. = __________ × __________ 100

= __________ % w/v

$$\% \text{ purity} = \frac{A}{E^{1\%}_{1\text{cm}}} \times \frac{\text{Avg. wt.}}{\text{L.C.}} \times \frac{100}{\text{D.F.}}$$

$$= \_\_\_\_\_\_ \times \_\_\_\_\_\_ \times \frac{100}{\_\_\_\_}$$

= __________ %

RESULT

The percentage purity of given sample of 0.04 gm of Propranolol HCl tablet I.P. was found to be __________%.

Flame Photometry 2

EXPERIMENT 2.1 A

Date ______________

ESTIMATION OF SODIUM CONCENTRATION IN GIVEN SAMPLE BY FLAME PHOTOMETRY

AIM

To determine the sodium concentration in the given sample.

PRINCIPLE

The technique of flame photometry is based upon the measurement of emitted radiations when a solution of metal compound is introduced into the flame in the form of droplets.

The fine residue forms the neutral atom which absorbs the energy from the flame and excites. While relaxing (ground state), these excited atoms emit the radiations. The wavelength of the emitted radiations is the characteristic of an element and can be used for qualitative analysis, while the intensity of the emitted radiations denote the concentration of the metal present in the solution.

The alkalies and alkaline earth metals such as Na, K, Li and Ca can be determined by flame photometry as the energy obtained by the flame is quite sufficient for the excitation of these elements.

Flame photometry is also known as flame emission spectroscopy because of the use of a flame to provide the energy of excitation to atoms introduced into the flame.

Flame photometry is a simple, rapid method for the routine analysis of metals of first two columns of the periodic table, but it is also successfully used for certain transition elements such as copper, iron and manganese.

The quantitative results can be obtained by plotting a calibration curve between the concentration of the element and flame intensity.

The processes involved in flame photometry are complex, but it should follow the following steps:

1. Liquid sample containing element, is aspirated into a flame to the formation of the liquid droplets.
2. Evaporation of liquid droplets, resulting formation of salt residue.
3. Then decomposition of residue to formation of free neutral atoms or radicals. These neutral atoms are excited by the thermal energy of the flame. The excited atoms which are unstable, quickly emit photons (radiation) and return to the lower energy state. The measurement of emitted radiation in terms of wavelength or intensity is basis of flame photometry.

If E_2 and E_1 represent the energy of the higher and lower energy state, the radiation emitted during the changing energy levels may be defined by equation as;

$$E_2 - E_1 = h\nu$$

Where h is the Planks constant, and ν is the frequency of emitted light which is defined as follows.

$$\nu = \frac{c}{\lambda}$$

we get,

$$E_2 - E_1 = hc/\lambda$$

or

$$\lambda = hc/E_2 - E_1$$

From the above equation, calculate the wavelength of the emitted radiation which is characteristic of the particular from which it was emitted.

PROCEDURE

1. Weigh accurately 100 mg of sodium chloride and dissolve in 100 ml of distilled water.
2. Take 10 ml of the solution and dilute to 100 ml with distilled water.
3. Prepare a series of standard solutions of 10, 20, 30, 40 and 50 μg/ml concentrations.
4. Switch on the flame photometer and select the sodium filter.
5. Set the gas in flame in order to get non-luminous flame and air pressure at 0.4 to 0.5 kg/cm^2.
6. Atomize the flame intensity to 0% using distilled water with the knob.
7. Atomize the flame intensity to 100% using 50 μg/ml standard solution (highest concentration).
8. Measure the per cent flame intensity of all the standard solutions (10 μg/ml, 20 μg/ml, 30 μg/ml, 40 μg/ml and 50 μg/ml concentration) and unknown sample solution.
9. Plot the graph between concentration and per cent flame intensity.
10. From the graph, mark the percentage flame intensity of the unknown sample and by extrapolating, determine the corresponding concentration.

Preparation of standard solution

100 mg standard in 100 ml water = 1 mg/ml = 1000 μg/ml

∴ 10 ml of 1 mg/ml diluted to100 ml water = 100 μg/ml

1 ml of 100 μg/ml diluted to 10 ml = 10 μg/ml

2 ml of 100 μg/ml diluted to 10 ml = 20 μg/ml

3 ml of 100 μg/ml diluted to 10 ml = 30 μg/ml

4 ml of 100 μg/ml diluted to 10 ml = 40 μg/ml

5 ml of 100 μg/ml diluted to 10 ml = 50 μg/ml

OBSERVATIONS

S. No.	Concentration (μg/ml)	Flame intensity (%)
1.	0	0
2.	10	19
3.	20	38
4.	30	59
5.	40	80
6.	50	100
7.	Unknown (Sample)	72

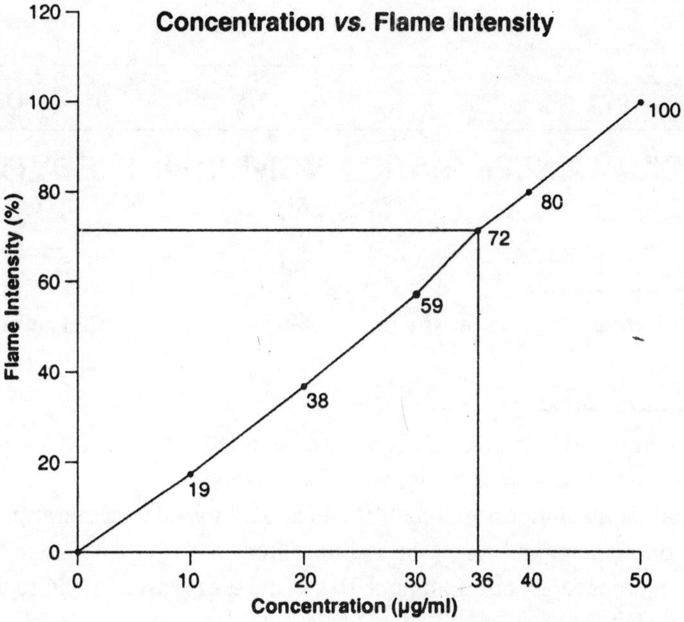

RESULT

The concentration of sodium ions in the given sample of NaCl solution was found to be 36 μg/ml by flame photometry.

EXPERIMENT 2.1 B

Date ______________

ESTIMATION OF SODIUM CONCENTRATION IN GIVEN SAMPLE BY FLAME PHOTOMETRY

(Manual)

AIM

To determine the sodium concentration in the given sample by flame photometry.

PROCEDURE

1. Weigh accurately 100 mg of sodium chloride and dissolve in 100 ml of distilled water.
2. Take 10 ml of the solution and dilute to 100 ml with distilled water.
3. Prepare a series of standard solutions of 10, 20, 30, 40 and 50 μg/ml concentrations.
4. Switch on the flame photometer and select the sodium filter.
5. Set the gas in flame in order to get non-luminous flame and air pressure at 0.4 to 0.5 kg/cm^2.
6. Atomize the flame intensity to 0% using distilled water with the knob.
7. Atomize the flame intensity to 100% using 50 μg/ml standard solution (highest concentration).
8. Measure the per cent flame intensity of all the standard solutions (10 μg/ml, 20 μg/ml, 30 μg/ml, 40 μg/ml and 50 μg/ml concentration) and unknown sample solution.
9. Plot the graph between concentration and per cent flame intensity.
10. From the graph, mark the percentage flame intensity of the unknown sample and by extrapolating, determine the corresponding concentration.

Preparation of standard solution:

100 mg standard in 100 ml water = 1 mg/ml = 1000 μg/ml

∴ 10 ml of 1mg/ml diluted to100 ml water = 100 μg/ml

1 ml of 100 μg/ml diluted to 10 ml = 10 μg/ml

2 ml of 100 μg/ml diluted to 10 ml = 20 μg/ml

3 ml of 100 μg/ml diluted to 10 ml = 30 μg/ml

4 ml of 100 μg/ml diluted to 10 ml = 40 μg/ml

5 ml of 100 μg/ml diluted to 10 ml = 50 μg/ml

OBSERVATIONS

S. No.	Concentration (μg/ml)	Flame intensity (%)
1.		
2.		
3.		
4.		
5.		
6.		
7.	Unknown (Sample)	

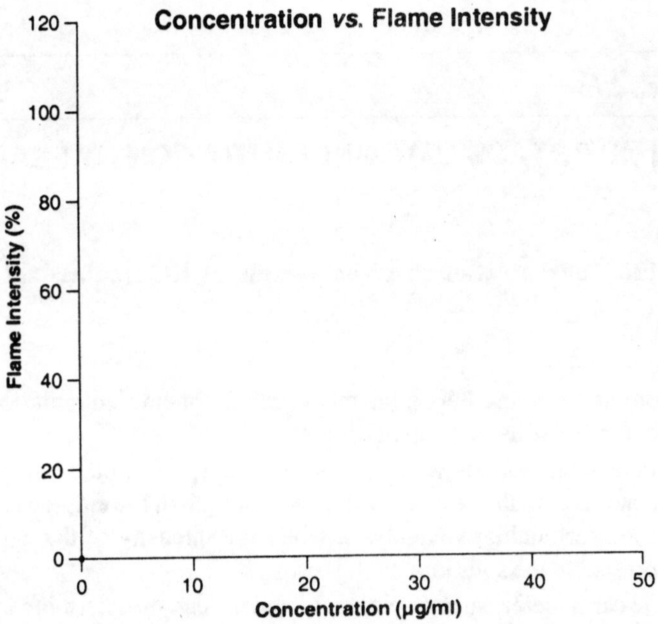

RESULT

The concentration of sodium ions in the given sample of NaCl solution was found to be __________ μg/ml by flame photometry.

EXPERIMENT 2.2A

Date ____________

DETERMINATION OF POTASSIUM CONCENTRATION BY FLAME PHOTOMETRY

AIM

To determine the potassium concentration in given sample of KCl (potassium chloride).

PRINCIPLE

The technique of flame photometry is based upon the measurement of emitted radiations when a solution of metal compound is introduced into the flame in the form of droplets.

The fine residue forms the neutral atoms which absorb the energy from the flame and excite. While relaxing (ground state), these excited atoms emit the radiations. The wavelength of the emitted radiations is the characteristic of an element and can be used for qualitative analysis, while the intensity of the emitted radiations denotes the concentration of the metal present in the solution.

The alkalies and alkaline earth metals such as Na, K, Li and Ca can be determined by flame photometry, as the energy obtained by the flame is quite sufficient for the excitation of these elements.

The quantitative results can be obtained by plotting a calibration curve between the concentration of the element and flame intensity.

PROCEDURE

1. Weigh accurately 100 mg of sodium chloride and dissolve in 100 ml of distilled water.
2. Take 10 ml of the solution and dilute to 100 ml with distilled water.
3. Prepare a series of standard solutions of 10, 20, 30, 40 and 50 μg/ml concentrations.
4. Switch on the flame photometer and select the Potassium filter.
5. Set the gas in flame in order to get non-luminous flame and air pressure at 0.4 to 0.5 kg/cm^2.
6. Atomize the flame intensity to 0% using distilled water with the knob.
7. Atomize the flame intensity to 100% using 50 μg/ml standard solution (highest concentration).
8. Measure the per cent flame intensity of all the standard solutions (10 μg/ml, 20 μg/ml, 30 μg/ml, 40 μg/ml and 50 μg/ml concentrations) and unknown sample solution.
9. Plot the graph between concentration and per cent flame intensity.
10. From the graph, mark the per cent flame intensity of the unknown sample and by extrapolating, determine the corresponding concentration.

OBSERVATIONS

S. No.	Concentrations (μg/ml)	Percentage of flame intensity
1.	0	0
2.	10	20
3.	20	39
4.	30	62
5.	40	81
6.	50	100
7.	Unknown (Sample)	57

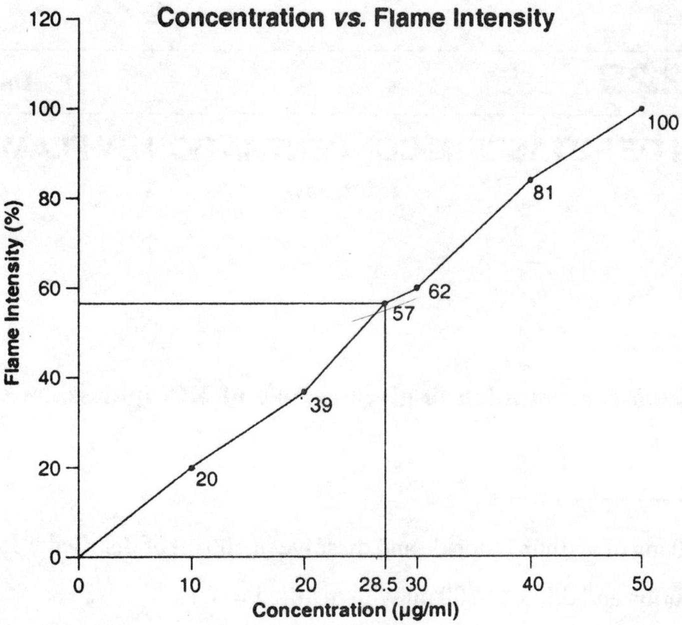

RESULT

The concentration of potassium ion in the given sample of KCl found to be 28.5 μg/ml by flame photometry.

EXPERIMENT 2.2B

Date ____________

DETERMINATION OF POTASSIUM CONCENTRATION BY FLAME PHOTOMETRY (Manual)

AIM

To determine the potassium concentration in given sample of KCl (potassium chloride).

PROCEDURE

1. Weigh accurately 100 mg of sodium chloride and dissolve in 100 ml of distilled water.
2. Take 10 ml of the solution and dilute to 100 ml with distilled water.
3. Prepare a series of standard solutions of 10, 20, 30, 40 and 50 μg/ml concentrations.
4. Switch on the flame photometer and select the Potassium filter.
5. Set the gas in flame in order to get non-luminous flame and air pressure at 0.4 to 0.5 kg/cm^2.
6. Atomize the flame intensity to 0%, using distilled water with the knob.
7. Atomize the flame intensity to 100%, using 50 μg/ml standard solution (highest concentration).
8. Measure the per cent flame intensity of all the standard solutions (10 μg/ml, 20 μg/ml, 30 μg/ml, 40 μg/ml and 50 μg/ml concentration) and unknown sample solution.
9. Plot the graph between concentration and per cent flame intensity.
10. From the graph, mark the per cent flame intensity of the unknown sample and by extrapolating, determine the corresponding concentration.

OBSERVATIONS

S. No.	Concentrations (μg/ml)	Percentage of flame intensity
1.	0	
2.	10	
3.	20	
4.	30	
5.	40	
6.	50	
7.	Unknown (Sample)	

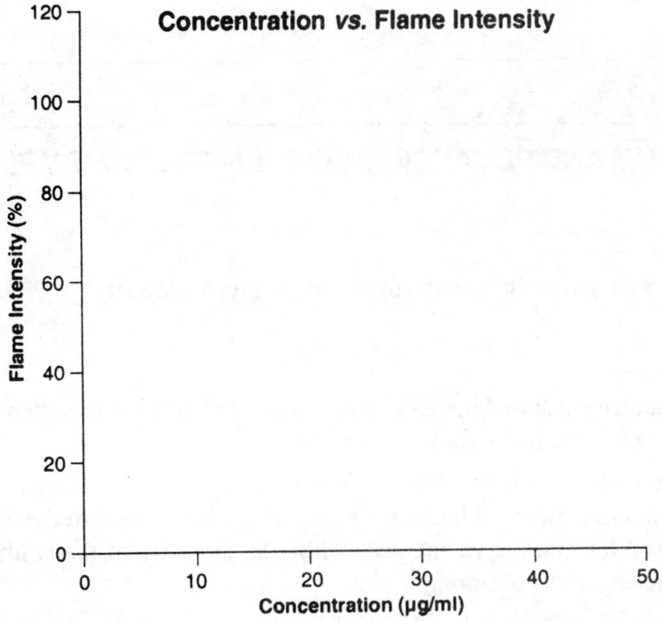

RESULT

The concentration of potassium ion in the given sample of KCl found to be __________ μg/ml by flame photometry.

EXPERIMENT 2.3 A

Date ______________

ESTIMATION OF SODIUM AND POTASSIUM CONCENTRATION BY FLAME PHOTOMETRY

AIM

To determine the sodium and potassium concentration in given sample.

PRINCIPLE

The technique of flame photometry is based upon the measurement of emitted radiations when a solution of metal compound is introduced into the flame in the form of droplets.

The fine residue forms the neutral atoms which absorb the energy from the flame and excite. While relaxing (ground state), these excited atoms emit the radiations. The wavelength of the emitted radiations is the characteristic of an element and can be used for qualitative analysis, while the intensity of the emitted radiations denotes the concentration of the metal present in the solution.

The alkalies and alkaline earth metals such as Na, K, Li and Ca can be determined by flame photometry, as the energy obtained by the flame is quite sufficient for the excitation of these elements.

The quantitative results can be obtained by plotting a calibration curve between the concentration of the element and flame intensity.

PROCEDURE

1. Prepare a series of standard solutions of 10, 20, 30, 40 and 50 µg/ml concentrations of NaCl and KCl separately.
2. Switch on the flame photometer and select the sodium filter.
3. Set the gas in flame in order to get non-luminous flame and air pressure at 0.4 to 0.5 kg/cm^2.
4. Atomize the flame intensity to 0% using distilled water with the knob.
5. Atomize the flame intensity to 100%, using 50 µg/ml standard solution (highest concentration).
6. Measure the per cent flame intensity of all the standard solutions (10 µg/ml, 20 µg/ml, 30 µg/ml, 40 µg/ml and 50 µg/ml concentration) and unknown sample solution.
7. Adopt the same procedure by selecting the potassium filter.
8. Plot the graph between concentration and per cent flame intensity with respect to sodium and potassium.
9. From the graph, mark the per cent flame intensity of the unknown sample and by extrapolating, determine the corresponding sodium and potassium concentration.

OBSERVATIONS

FOR SODIUM

S. No.	Concentration (µg/ml)	% flame intensity
1.	0	0
2.	10	19
3.	20	38
4.	30	59
5.	40	80
6.	50	100
7.	Unknown (Sample)	78

FOR POTASSIUM

S. No.	Concentration (µg/ml)	% flame intensity
1.	0	0
2.	10	20
3.	20	39
4.	30	56
5.	40	80
6.	50	100
7.	Unknown (sample)	66

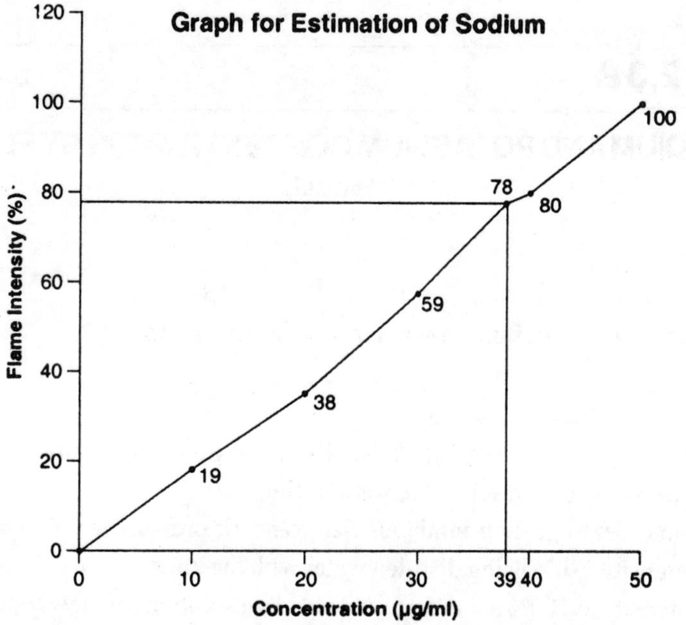

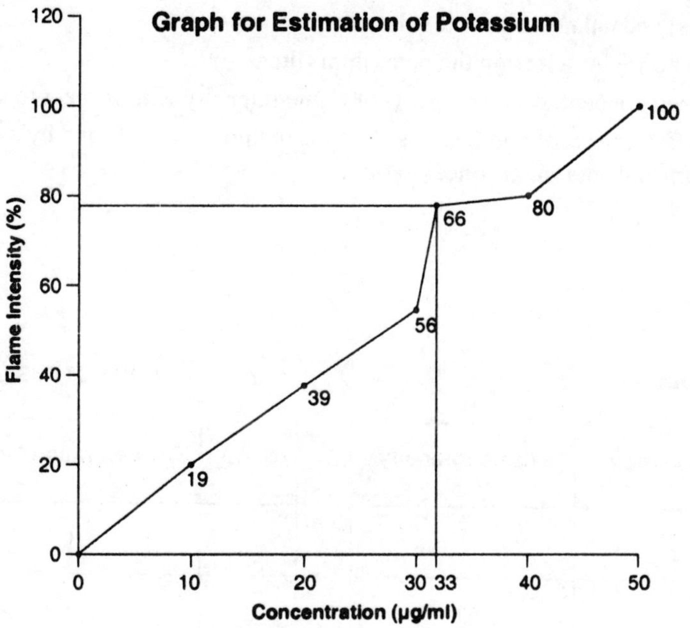

RESULT

The concentration of sodium and potassium in the given sample was found to be 39 µg/ml and 33 µg/ml by flame photometry respectively.

EXPERIMENT 2.3B

Date ____________

ESTIMATION OF SODIUM AND POTASSIUM CONCENTRATION BY FLAME PHOTOMETRY (Manual)

AIM

To determine the sodium and potassium concentration in given sample.

PROCEDURE

1. Prepare a series of standard solutions of 10, 20, 30, 40 and 50 µg/ml concentrations of NaCl and KCl.
2. Switch on the flame photometer and select the sodium filter.
3. Set the gas in flame in order to get non-luminous flame and air pressure at 0.4 to 0.5 kg/cm^2.
4. Atomize the flame intensity to 0% using distilled water with the knob.
5. Atomize the flame intensity to 100% using 50 µg/ml standard solution (highest concentration).
6. Measure the per cent flame intensity of all the standard solutions (10 µg/ml, 20 µg/ml, 30 µg/ml, 40 µg/ml and 50 µg/ml concentrations) and unknown sample solution.
7. Adopt the same procedure by selecting the potassium filter.
8. Plot the graph between concentration and per cent flame intensity with respect to sodium and potassium.
9. From the graph, mark the per cent flame intensity of the unknown sample and by extrapolating, determine the corresponding sodium and potassium concentration.

OBSERVATIONS

FOR SODIUM

S. No.	Concentration (µg/ml)	% flame intensity
1.		
2.		
3.		
4.		
5.		
6.		
7.	Unknown (Sample)	

FOR POTASSIUM

S. No.	Concentration (µg/ml)	% flame intensity
1.		
2.		
3.		
4.		
5.		
6.		
7.	Unknown (sample)	

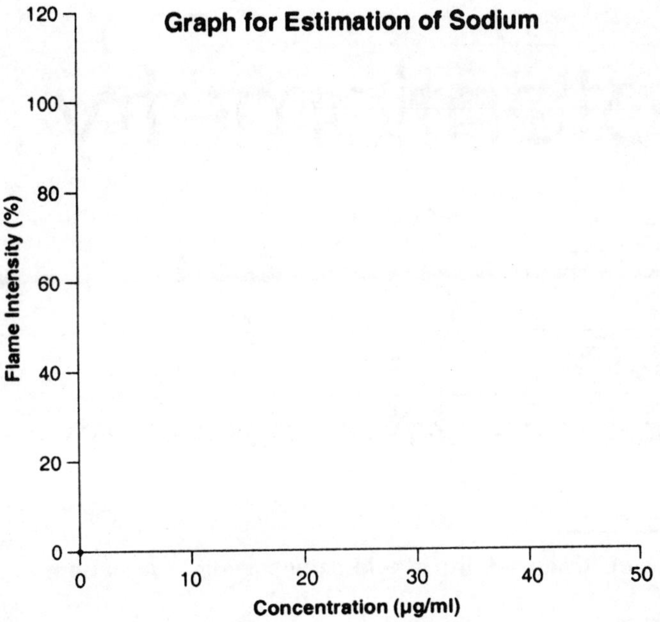

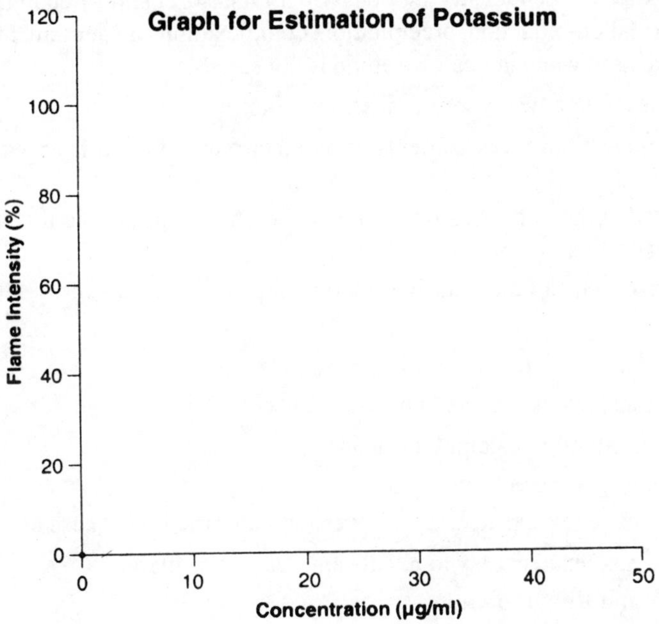

RESULT

The concentration of sodium and potassium in the given sample was found to be ______ µg/ml and ________ µg/ml by flame photometry respectively.

Potentiometry

3

EXPERIMENT 3.1 A

Date ________________

DETERMINATION OF STRENGTH OF STRONG ACID BY POTENTIOMETRY

AIM

To determine the strength of strong sulphuric acid using strong base sodium hydroxide by potentiometry.

PRINCIPLE

Potentiometry is a branch of electrochemistry that deals with measurement of changes in the electrode potential (e.m.f.) which involve in oxidation-reduction, precipitation, complexation and neutralization equilibria reactions. The potentiometric titrations are used when indicator method is not suitable.

Potentiometric methods include two types of measurements:

1. **Direct method:** In this method measurements of an electrode potential from which the concentration of an active ion may be found.
2. **Indirect method:** In this method measurements by the change in potential (e.m.f.) of an electrolytic cell brought about by the addition of a titrant.

Above methods are based on the quantitative relationship of the e.m.f. of a cell as given by the following equation:

$$E_{\text{cell}} = E_{\text{reference}} + E_{\text{indicator}} + E_{\text{junction}}$$

In potentiometric titrations, two types of electrodes are used:

(*a*) Indicator electrode e.g. saturated calomel electrode

(*b*) Reference electrode e.g. glass electrode

Potentiometric titration have several advantages over indicator method. These are:

1. The apparatus used is inexpensive, easy to handle and readily available.
2. It is used for coloured and dilute solutions.
3. Results are easy to interpret.
4. Several components can be titrated in the same reaction cell.

PROCEDURE

1. Switch on the potentiometer.
2. Connect the calomel electrode to positive terminal and the glass electrode to negative terminal.
3. Rinse the electrodes with distilled water.
4. Set the temperature knob at room temperature.
5. Calibrate the electrodes by using standard buffer solution of pH 7.0 and pH 9.2.

6. Set the function key to pH position using standard buffer solution and adjust pH value to 7 by the calibration control knob.
7. Again check by using the second buffer solution at pH 9.2.
8. Rinse the beaker and electrodes with distilled water thoroughly.
9. Immerse the electrodes in 50 ml of H_2SO_4 (1N approx.) and note the e.m.f. in mV (millivolt) reading.
10. Switch on the stirrer.
11. Add 1 ml of 1N NaOH at a time and note the mV readings.
12. Take several readings before and after the approx. end point.
13. Plot the graph between
    (*a*) Normal curve, i.e. e.m.f *vs.* Volume of NaOH.
    (*b*) 1st derivative curve, i.e. $\Delta\varepsilon/\Delta V$ *vs.* Volume of NaOH.
    (*c*) 2nd derivative curve, i.e. $\Delta^2\varepsilon/\Delta V^2$ *vs.* Volume of NaOH.

OBSERVATION TABLE

S. No.	Vol. of NaOH (ml)	e.m.f. (mV)	$\frac{\Delta\varepsilon}{\Delta V} = \frac{\varepsilon_2 - \varepsilon_1}{V_2 - V_1}$	$\frac{\Delta^2\varepsilon}{\Delta V^L}$
1.	0	294	– 2	1
2.	1	292	– 1	– 3
3.	2	291	– 4	– 2
4.	3	287	– 6	1
5.	4	281	– 5	– 3
6.	5	276	– 8	– 6
7.	6	268	– 14	– 20
8.	7	254	– 34	– 490
9.	8	220	– 524	504
10.	9	– 304	– 14	– 1
11.	10	– 318	– 15	10
12.	11	– 333	– 5	
13.	12	– 338		

Normal Curve: Vol. of NaOH *vs.* e.m.f.

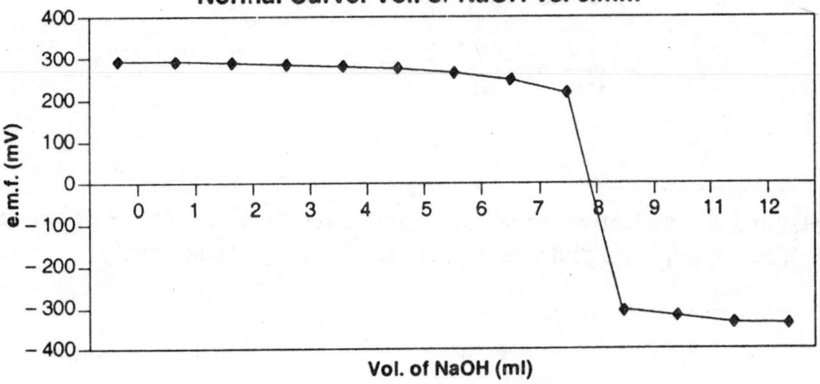

First Derivative Curve: Vol. of NaOH *vs.* e.m.f.

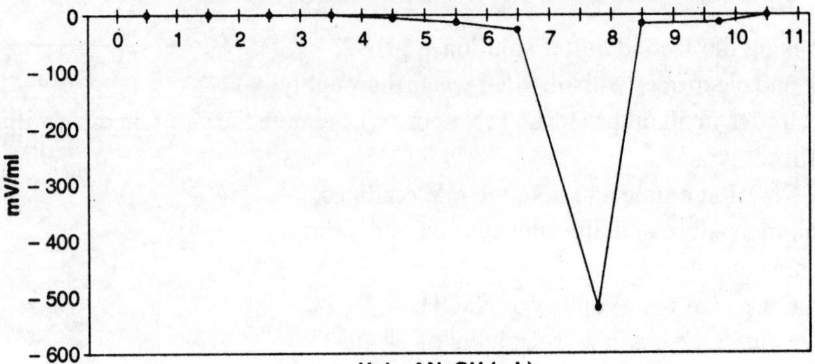

Second Derivative Curve: Vol. of NaOH *vs.* e.m.f.

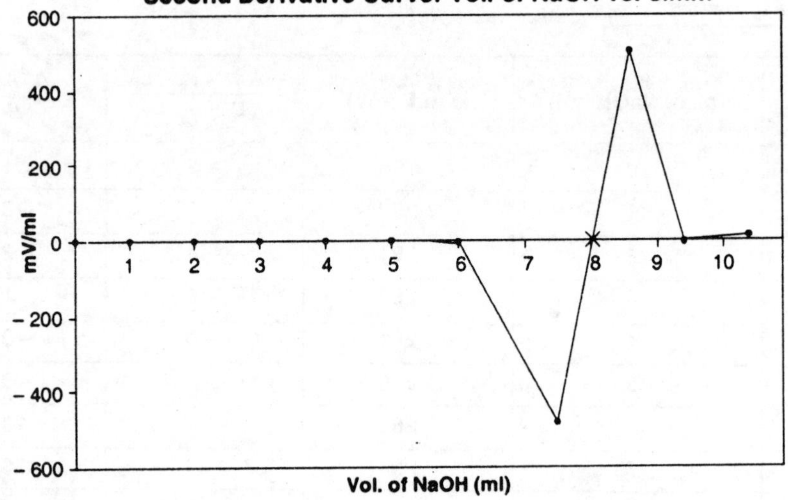

From the second derivative graph

Volume of NaOH = 7.5 ml

Formula

$$? = N_1 = \text{Normality of } H_2SO_4 \text{ to be calculated}$$

$$50 \text{ ml} = V_1 = \text{Volume of acid taken}$$

$$1 \text{ N} = N_2 = \text{Normality of NaOH}$$

$$7.5 \text{ ml} = V_2 = \text{Volume of NaOH (from graph)}$$

$$N_1 = \frac{N_2 \times V_2}{V_1} = \frac{1 \times 7.5}{50} = 0.15 \text{ N}$$

RESULT

The normal curve, 1st and 2nd derivative curves were plotted for the given sample of strong sulphuric acid. The normality of the given strong sulphuric acid was found to be 0.15 N by potentiometry.

EXPERIMENT 3.1 B

Date ______________

DETERMINATION OF STRENGTH OF STRONG ACID BY POTENTIOMETRY
(Manual)

AIM

To determine the strength of strong acid (sulphuric acid) using strong base sodium hydroxide by potentiometry.

PROCEDURE

1. Switch on the potentiometer.
2. Connect the calomel electrode to positive terminal and the glass electrode to negative terminal.
3. Rinse the electrodes with distilled water.
4. Set the temperature knob at room temperature.
5. Calibrate the electrodes by using standard buffer solution of pH 7.0 and pH 9.2.
6. Set the function key to pH position using standard buffer solution and adjust pH value to 7 by the calibration control knob.
7. Again check by using the second buffer solution at pH 9.2.
8. Rinse the beaker and electrodes with distilled water thoroughly.
9. Immerse the electrodes in 50 ml of H_2SO_4 (1N approx.) and note the e.m.f. in mV (millivolt) reading.
10. Switch on the stirrer.
11. Add 1 ml of 1N NaOH at a time and note the mV readings.
12. Take several readings before and after the approx. end point.
13. Plot the graph between:
    (*a*) Normal curve, i.e. e.m.f. *vs*. volume of NaOH.
    (*b*) 1st derivative curve, i.e. $\Delta\varepsilon/\Delta V$ *vs*. volume of NaOH.
    (*c*) 2nd derivative curve, i.e. $\Delta^2\varepsilon/\Delta V^2$ *vs*. volume of NaOH

OBSERVATION TABLE

S. No.	Vol. of NaOH (ml)	e.m.f. (mV)	$\frac{\Delta\varepsilon}{\Delta V} = \frac{\varepsilon_2 - \varepsilon_1}{V_2 - V_1}$	$\frac{\Delta^2\varepsilon}{\Delta V^L}$
1.	0			
2.	1			
3.	2			
4.	3			
5.	4			
6.	5			
7.	6			

(Contd.)

S. No.	Vol. of NaOH (ml)	e.m.f. (mV)	$\frac{\Delta \varepsilon}{\Delta V} = \frac{\varepsilon_2 - \varepsilon_1}{V_2 - V_1}$	$\frac{\Delta^2 \varepsilon}{\Delta V^L}$
8.	7			
9.	8			
10.	9			
11.	10			
12.	11			
13.	12			

Normal Curve: Vol. of NaOH *vs.* e.m.f.

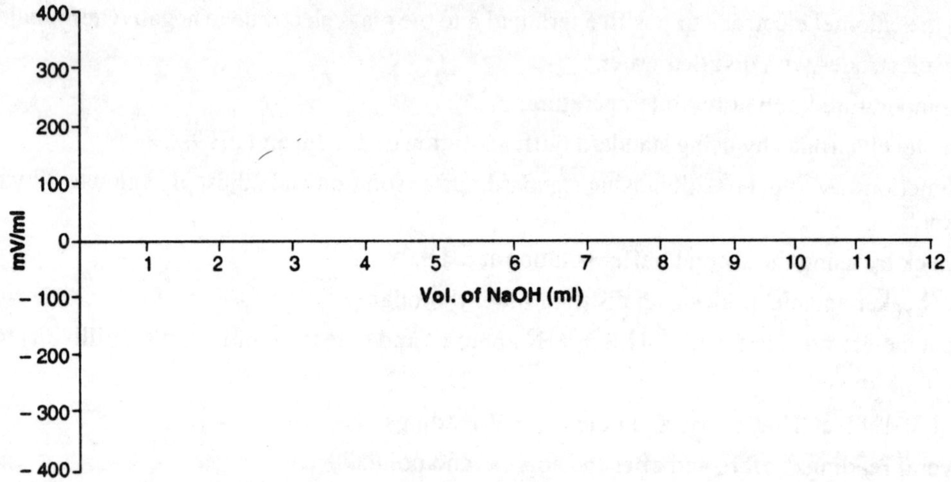

First Derivative Curve: Vol. of NaOH *vs.* e.m.f.

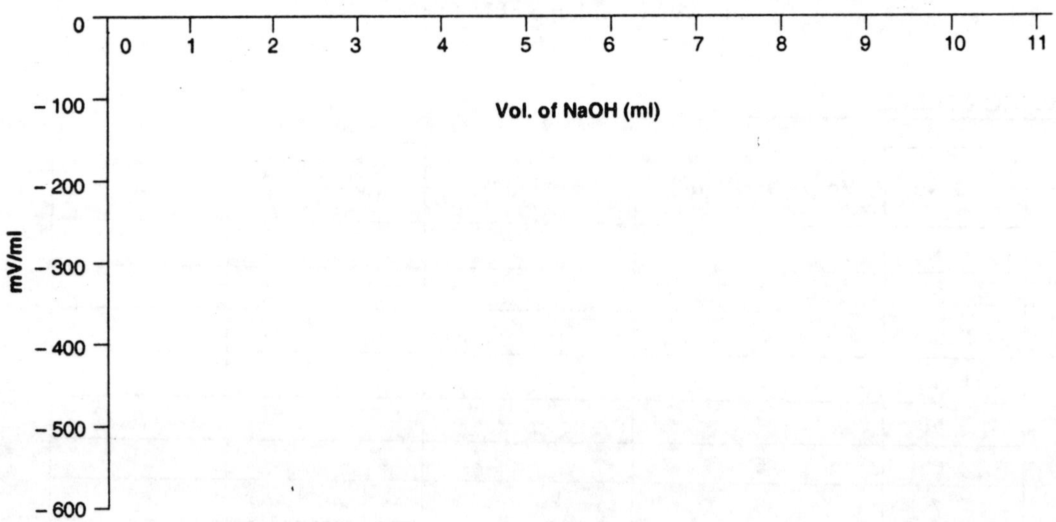

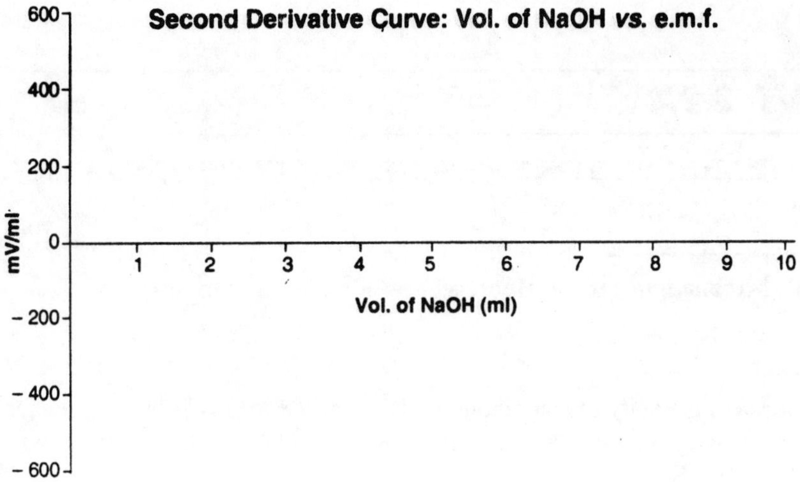

From the second derivative graph

Volume of NaOH = ___________ml

FORMULA

? = N_1 = **Normality of H_2SO_4 to be calculated**

50 ml = V_1 = **Volume of acid taken**

1N = N_2 = **Normality of NaOH**

___________ ml = V_2 = **Volume of NaOH (from graph)**

RESULT

The normal curve, 1st and 2nd derivative curves were plotted for the given sample of strong Sulphuric acid. The normality of the given strong Sulphuric acid was found to be ___________N by potentiometry.

EXPERIMENT 3.2 A

Date ______________

EFFECT OF QUENCHING ON THE FLUORESCENCE OF QUININE SULPHATE

AIM

To study the effect of quenching on the fluorescence of quinine sulphate.

PRINCIPLE

The reduction in fluorescent intensity of a compound due to certain ions is known as quenching. This decrease in fluorescent intensity may be due to various factors like pH, concentration, temperature, viscosity and presence of specific chemical substances (KI).

Quenching mainly is of four types:

1. Self quenching
2. Chemical quenching
3. Collisional quenching
4. Static quenching

The principle behind this experiment is the presence of halides (Iodide ions) leads to quenching due to collision.

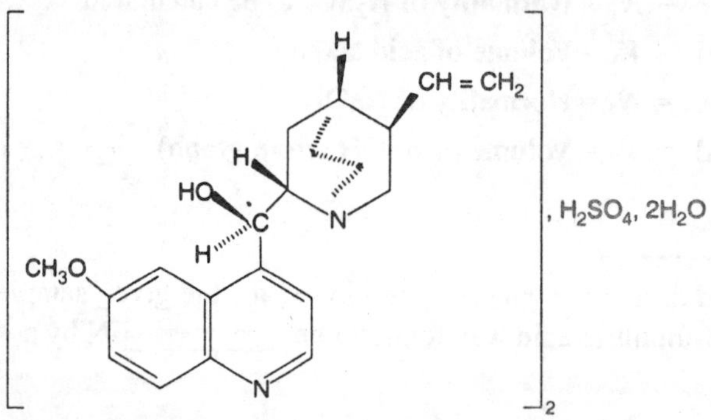

Mol. Formula: $(C_{20}H_{24}N_2O_2)_2,H_2SO_4,2H_2O$ **Mol. Wt.:** 782.95

Quinine sulphate is (8*S*, 9*R*)-6′-methoxycinchonan-9-ol sulphate dihydrate. The alkaloid is obtained from the bark of various species of Cinchona.

Category: Antimalarial.

Description: White or almost white, needle-like crystals or crystalline powder.

Solubility: Freely soluble in a mixture of 2 volumes of chloroform and 1 volume of ethanol; sparingly soluble in boiling water and in ethanol (95%); slightly soluble in water; very slightly soluble in chloroform; practically insoluble in ether.

ASSAY

Weigh accurately about 0.2 g, dissolve in a mixture of 10 ml of chloroform and 20 ml of acetic anhydride and carry out method A for non-aqueous titration as per I.P. 1996 (Appendix 3.45) determining the end-point potentiometrically. Perform a blank determination and make any necessary correction.

Each ml of 0.1M perchloric acid is equivalent to 0.02490 g of $(C_{20}H_{24}N_2O_2)_2$, H_2SO_4.

USES

Antimalarial.

PROCEDURE

1. **Preparation of Quinine sulphate solution**
   (*a*) Take 100 mg of Quinine sulphate and dissolve in 100 ml of 0.1N H_2SO_4 (1 mg/ml).
   (*b*) Take 10 ml of the solution and dilute to 100 ml with 0.1N H_2SO_4 (100 μg/ml).
   (*c*) Again 10 ml of this solution dilute to 100 ml with 0.1N H_2SO_4 (10 μg/ml).
   (*d*) For final concentration, take 10 ml of the above solution and dilute to 100 ml with 0.1N H_2SO_4 (1 μg/ml).
2. **Preparation of KI solution**
   (*a*) Dissolve 100 mg of KI in 100 ml of 0.1N H_2SO_4 (1 mg/ml).
   (*b*) Dilute 10 ml of above solution to 100 ml with 0.1N H_2SO_4 (100 μg/ml).
3. In six 10 ml volumetric flasks, take 1 ml of 1 μg/ml solution in each.
4. Add 1, 2, 3, 4 and 5 ml of KI solution in each flask.
5. Make up the volume to 10 ml with 0.1N H_2SO_4.
6. Set the flame intensity to zero percent using 0.1N H_2SO_4 as blank and 100% using standard solution (not containing KI).
7. Plot the graph between volume of KI added and % F.I.

OBSERVATIONS

S. No.	Volume of KI added (ml)	% F.I.
1.	0	100
2.	1.00	40
3.	2.00	33
4.	3.00	24
5.	4.00	16
6.	5.00	08

Vol. of KI *vs.* Fluorescence Intensity

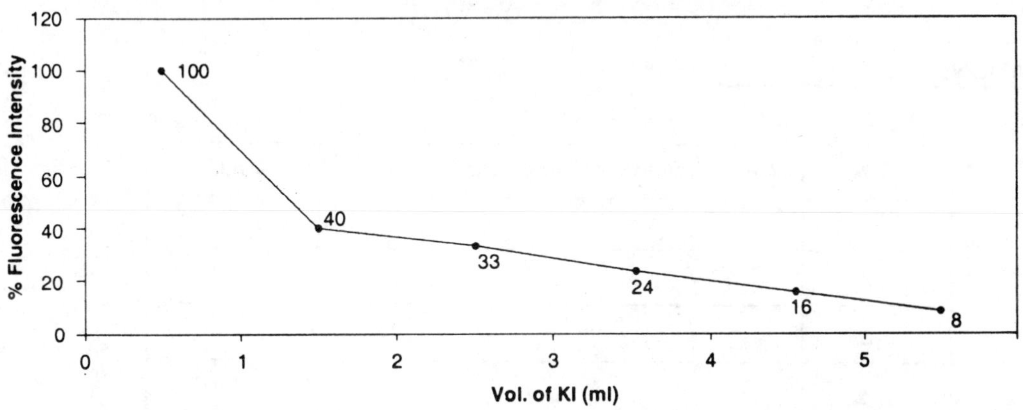

RESULT

A decrease in fluorescent intensity was observed for quinine sulphate with the addition of potassium iodide solution.

EXPERIMENT 3.2B

Date ____________

EFFECT OF QUENCHING ON THE FLUORESCENCE OF QUININE SULPHATE

(Manual)

AIM

To study the effect of quenching on the fluorescence of quinine sulphate.

PROCEDURE

1. **Preparation of Quinine sulphate solution**
   (*a*) Take 100 mg of Quinine sulphate and dissolve in 100 ml of 0.1N H_2SO_4 (1 mg/ml).
   (*b*) Take 10 ml of the solution and dilute to 100 ml with 0.1N H_2SO_4 (100 μg/ml).
   (*c*) Again 10 ml of this solution dilute to 100 ml with 0.1N H_2SO_4 (10 μg/ml).
   (*d*) For final concentration, take 10 ml of the above solution and dilute to 100 ml with 0.1N H_2SO_4 (1 μg/ml).
2. **Preparation of KI solution**
   (*a*) Dissolve 100 mg of KI in 100 ml of 0.1N H_2SO_4 (1 mg/ml).
   (*b*) Dilute 10 ml of above solution to 100 ml with 0.1N H_2SO_4 (100 μg/ml).
3. In six 10 ml volumetric flasks, take 1 ml of 1 μg/ml solution in each.
4. Add 1, 2, 3, 4 and 5 ml of KI solution in each flask.
5. Make up the volume to 10 ml with 0.1N H_2SO_4.
6. Set the flame intensity to zero percent using 0.1N H_2SO_4 as blank and 100% using standard solution (not containing KI).
7. Plot the graph between volume of KI added and % F.I.

OBSERVATIONS

S. No.	Volume of KI added (ml)	% F.I.
1.		
2.		
3.		
4.		
5.		
6.		

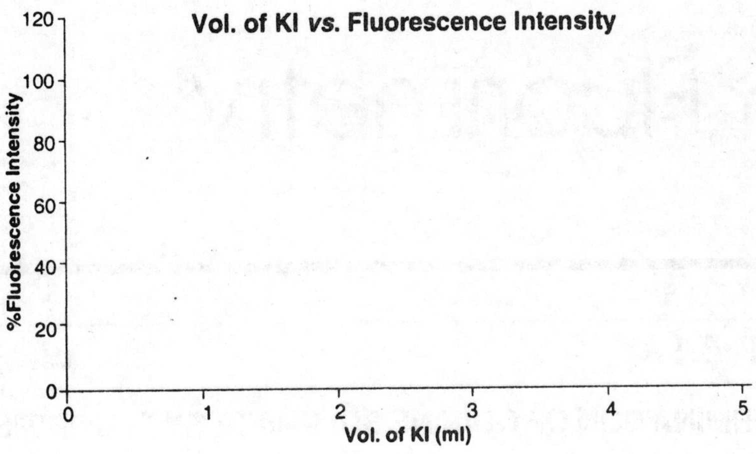

RESULT

A decrease in fluorescent intensity was observed for quinine sulphate with the addition of potassium iodide solution.

Fluorimetry

4

EXPERIMENT 4.1 A

Date ____________

DETERMINATION OF QUININE SULPHATE BY FLUORIMETRY

AIM

To determine the concentration of quinine sulphate by fluorimetry.

PRINCIPLE

When any molecule absorbs U.V./visible radiation, its electrons transmit from singlet ground state to singlet excited state and as this excited state is not stable, it emits the radiation and returns to stable singlet ground state. This phenomenon of emission of radiation is known as fluorescence. The fluorimetry is the measurement of this emitted radiation.

The emitted radiation (fluorescent intensity) is directly proportional to the concentration of substance present, which can be measured by fluorimeter.

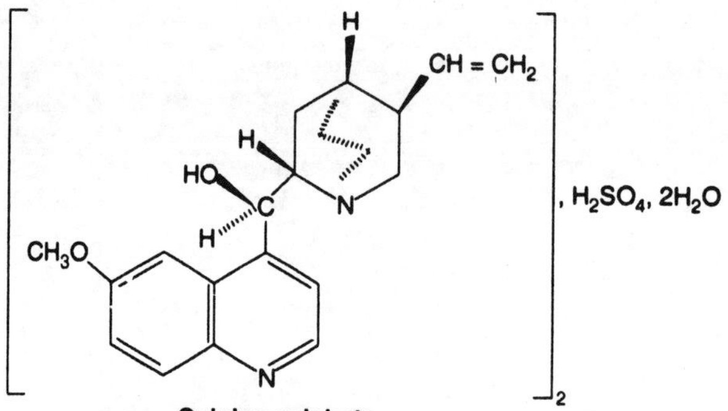

Quinine sulphate

Mol. Formula: $(C_{20}H_{24}N_2O_2)_2$, H_2SO_4, $2H_2O$ **Mol. Wt.:** 782.95

Quinine sulphate is (8S, 9R)-6′-methoxycinchonan-9-ol sulphate dihydrate. The alkaloid is obtained from the bark of various species of cinchona.

Category: Antimalarial.

Description: White or almost white, needle-like crystals or crystalline powder.

Solubility: Freely soluble in a mixture of 2 volumes of chloroform and 1 volume of ethanol; sparingly soluble in boiling water and in ethanol (95%); slightly soluble in water; very slightly soluble in chloroform; practically insoluble in ether.

ASSAY

Weigh accurately about 0.2 g, dissolve in a mixture of 10 ml of chloroform and 20 ml of acetic anhydride and carry out method A as per I.P. 1996 (Appendix 3.45) for non-aqueous titration determining the end-point potentiometrically. Perform a blank determination and make any necessary correction.

Each ml of 0.1M perchloric acid is equivalent to 0.02490 g of $(C_{20}H_{24}N_2O_2)_2$, H_2SO_4.

PROCEDURE

1. **Preparation of standard solution**
   (*a*) Weigh accurately 100 mg of Quinine sulphate powdered drug.
   (*b*) Dissolve in 100 ml of 0.1N H_2SO_4 (1 mg/ml).
   (*c*) Take 10 ml of above solution and dilute to 100 ml with 0.1N H_2SO_4 (100 μg/ml).
   (*d*) Again 10 ml of above solution dilute to 100 ml with 0.1N H_2SO_4 (10 μg/ml).
   (*e*) To get the resulting solution of 0.5, 1.0, 1.5, 2.0 and 2.5 μg/ml concentrations, take 0.5, 1.0, 1.5, 2.0 and 2.5 ml of above solutions respectively and dilute to 10 ml with 0.1N H_2SO_4.
2. **Preparation of sample solution**
   Pipette out 1 ml of given unknown sample solution and make up the volume to 10 ml with 0.1N H_2SO_4.
3. Switch on the instrument set the excitation and emission filters at the wavelengths 365 and 459 respectively.
4. Set the fluorescence intensity to 0% by using 0.1N H_2SO_4 as blank and 100% by using highest concentration of the standard solution (2.5 μg/ml).
5. Repeat the same at least for two times more to minimize the instrumental error.
6. Measure the percentage fluorescence intensity of different standard and sample solutions.
7. Plot a graph between concentrations *vs.* F.I. and determine the concentration of unknown sample by extrapolating the found F.I.

OBSERVATIONS

S. No.	Concentration (μg/ml)	% F.I.
1	0	0
2	0.5	20
3	1.0	42
4	1.5	61
5	2.0	79
6	2.5	100
7	Unknown	70

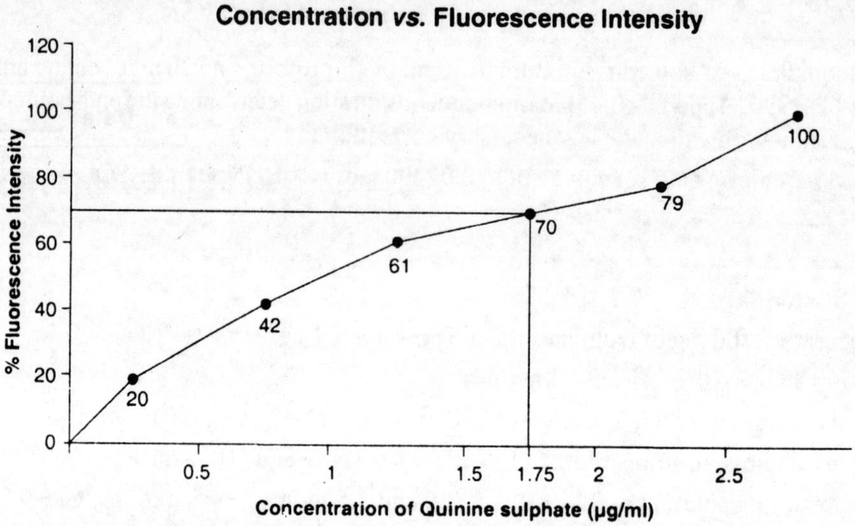

From graph the concentration of unknown solution = 1.75 μg/ml.

Since we have diluted the sample solution 10 times, so the concentration of quinine sulphate = 1.75 × 10 = 17.5 μg/ml.

RESULT

The concentration of the given sample of quinine sulphate was found to be 17.5 μg/ml by fluorimetry.

EXPERIMENT 4.1 B

Date ______________

DETERMINATION OF QUININE SULPHATE BY FLUORIMETRY
(Manual)

AIM

To determine the concentration of quinine sulphate by fluorimetry.

PROCEDURE

1. **Preparation of standard solution**
   (*a*) Weigh accurately 100 mg of Quinine sulphate powdered drug.
   (*b*) Dissolve in 100 ml of 0.1N H_2SO_4 (1 mg/ml).
   (*c*) Take 10 ml of above solution and dilute to 100 ml with 0.1N H_2SO_4 (100 μg/ml).
   (*d*) Again 10 ml of above solution dilute to 100 ml with 0.1N H_2SO_4 (10 μg/ml).
   (*e*) To get the resulting solution of 0.5, 1.0, 1.5, 2.0 and 2.5 μg/ml concentrations, take 0.5, 1.0, 1.5, 2.0 and 2.5 ml of above solutions respectively and dilute to 10 ml with 0.1N H_2SO_4.
2. **Preparation of sample solution**
   Pipette out 1 ml of given unknown sample solution and make up the volume to 10 ml with 0.1N H_2SO_4.
3. Switch on the instrument. Set the excitation and emission filters at the wavelengths 365 and 459 respectively.
4. Set the fluorescence intensity to 0% by using 0.1N H_2SO_4 as blank and 100% by using highest concentration of the standard solution (2.5 μg/ml).
5. Repeat the same at least for two times more to minimize the instrumental error.
6. Measure the percentage fluorescence intensity of different standard and sample solutions.
7. Plot a graph between concentrations *vs.* F.I. and determine the concentration of unknown sample by extrapolating the found F.I.

OBSERVATIONS

S. No.	Concentration (μg/ml)	% F.I.
1.	0	
2.	0.5	
3.	1.0	
4.	1.5	
5.	2.0	
6.	2.5	
7.	Unknown	

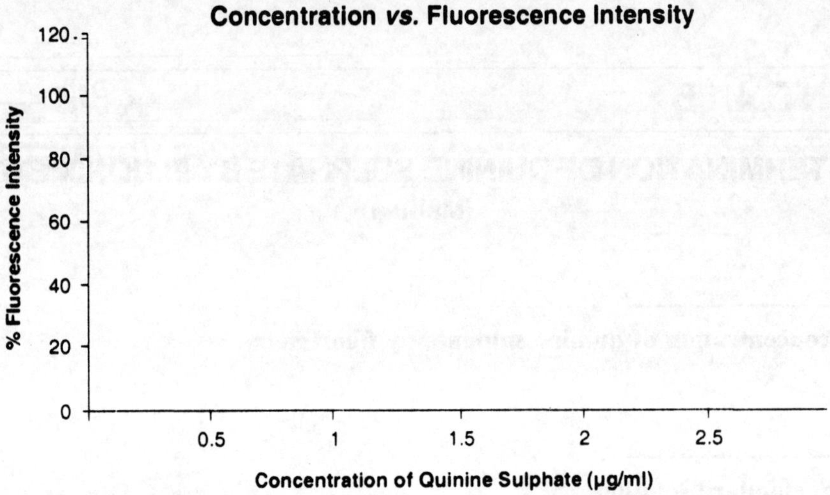

From graph, the concentration of unknown solution = __________ μg/ml.

Since we have diluted the sample solution 10 times so the concentration of quinine sulphate = _______ μg/ml.

RESULT

The concentration of the given sample of quinine sulphate was found to be __________ μg/ml by fluorimetry.

EXPERIMENT 4.2A

Date ______________

ASSAY OF QUININE SULPHATE TABLET BY FLUORIMETRY

AIM

To perform the assay of quinine sulphate tablet by fluorimetry.

PRINCIPLE

When any molecule absorbs U.V./visible radiation, its electrons transmit from singlet ground state to singlet excited state and as this excited state is not stable, it emits the radiation and returns to stable singlet ground state. This phenomenon of emission of radiation is known as fluorescence. The fluorimetry is the measurement of this emitted radiation.

The emitted radiation (fluorescent intensity) is directly proportional to the concentration of substance present, which can be measured by fluorimeter.

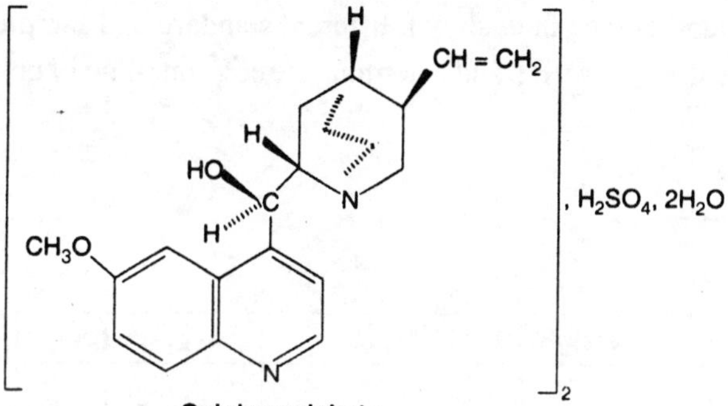

Quinine sulphate

Mol. Formula: $(C_{20}H_{24}N_2O_2)_2$, H_2SO_4, $2H_2O$ **Mol. Wt.:** 782.95

Quinine sulphate is (8S, 9R)-6′-methoxycinchonan-9-ol sulphate dihydrate. The alkaloid is obtained from the bark of various species of cinchona.

Category: Antimalarial.

Description: White or almost white, needle-like crystals or crystalline powder.

Solubility: Freely soluble in a mixture of 2 volumes of chloroform and 1 volume of ethanol; sparingly soluble in boiling water and in ethanol (95%); slightly soluble in water; very slightly soluble in chloroform; practically insoluble in ether.

ASSAY

Weigh accurately about 0.2 g, dissolve in a mixture of 10 ml of chloroform and 20 ml of acetic anhydride and carry out method A as per I.P. 1996 (Appendix 3.45) for non-aqueous titration determining the end-point potentiometrically. Perform a blank determination and make any necessary correction. Each ml of 0.1M perchloric acid is equivalent to 0.02490 g of $(C_{20}H_{24}N_2O_2)_2$, H_2SO_4.

PROCEDURE

1. **Preparation of standard solution**
   (*a*) Weigh accurately 100 mg of Quinine sulphate powdered drug.
   (*b*) Dissolve in 100 ml of 0.1N H_2SO_4 (1 mg/ml).
   (*c*) Take 10 ml of above solution and dilute to 100 ml with 0.1N H_2SO_4 (100 μg/ml).

(*d*) Again 10 ml of above solution dilute to 100 ml with 0.1N H_2SO_4 (10 μg/ml).

(*e*) To get the resulting solution of 0.5, 1.0, 1.5, 2.0 and 2.5 μg/ml concentrations, take 0.5, 1.0, 1.5, 2.0 and 2.5 ml of above solutions respectively and dilute to 10 ml with 0.1N H_2SO_4.

2. **Preparation of sample (Quinine sulphate tablets)**

(*a*) Weigh accurately 20 tablets and calculate the average weight.

(*b*) Powder the tablets and weigh accurately the powdered quantity equivalent to 100 mg of quinine sulphate.

(*c*) Dissolve in 75 ml of 0.1N H_2SO_4 by thorough mixing.

(*d*) Make up the volume to 100 ml with 0.1N H_2SO_4 and filter.

(*e*) Dilute 10 ml of above solution to 100 ml with 0.1N H_2SO_4.

(*f*) Again take 10 ml of the solution and dilute to 100 ml with 0.1 N H_2SO_4.

(*g*) To reach final concentration take 10 ml of the resulting solution and dilute to 100 ml to produce the concentration of 1 μg/ml.

3. Switch on the instrument. Set the excitation and emission filters at the wavelengths 365 and 459 respectively.
4. Set the fluorescence intensity to 0% by using 0.1N H_2SO_4 as blank and 100% by using highest concentration of the standard solution (2.5 μg/ml).
5. Repeat the same at least for two times more to minimize the instrumental error.
6. Measure the percentage fluorescence intensity of different standard and sample solutions.
7. Plot a graph between concentrations *vs.* F.I. and determine the concentration of unknown sample by extrapolating the found F.I.

OBSERVATIONS

1. **Weight variation test**

S. No.	Weight of tablet (gm)	Avg. wt. (gm)
1.	0.365	0.380
2.	0.380	
3.	0.375	
4.	0.386	
5.	0.374	
6.	0.379	
7.	0.381	
8.	0.376	
9.	0.380	
10.	0.384	
11.	0.377	
12.	0.380	
13.	0.383	
14.	0.380	
15.	0.379	
16.	0.380	
17.	0.381	
18.	0.378	
19.	0.380	
20.	0.382	

2. Observation table

S. No.	Concentration%	% F.I.
1.	0	0
2.	0.5	20
3.	1.0	42
4.	1.5	60
5.	2.0	79
6.	2.5	100
7.	Sample	50

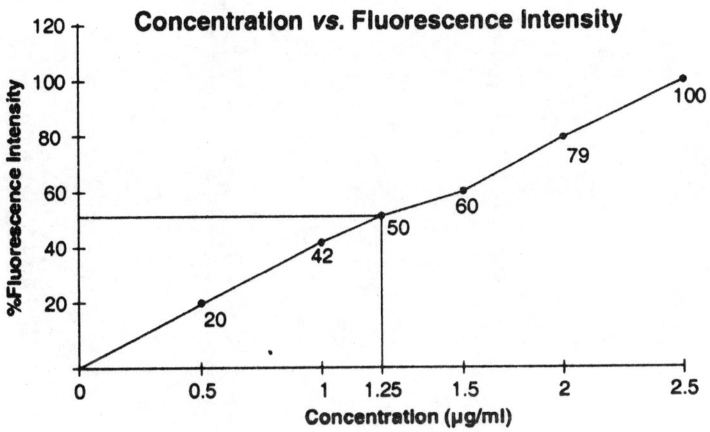

3. From graph, the concentration of Quinine sulphate drug = 1.25 μg/ml

CALCULATIONS

(*i*) Label claim of given tablet = 0.300 gm of Q.S.

(*ii*) Wt. of 20 tablets = 7.6 gm

(*iii*) Avg. wt. of each tablet = 0.380 gm

0.380 gm of powder contain = 0.300 gm of Q.S.

∴ x gm of powder = 0.100 gm of Q.S.

$$\therefore \quad x = \frac{0.380 \times 0.1}{0.3}$$

$$= \mathbf{0.126\ gm}$$

CALCULATIONS

(*i*) From graph, initial quantity of drug that would be present in dilution

$$= 1.25 \times \frac{100}{10} \times \frac{100}{10} \times \frac{100}{10} \times 100$$

$$= 0.125 \text{ gm/100 ml}$$

(*ii*) $\because$ 0.126 gm of powder = 0.125 gm of Quinine sulphate

$\therefore$ 0.380 gm of powder will contain $= \dfrac{0.125}{0.126} \times 0.380$

= 0.376 gm of Quinine sulphate

Practical value = 0.376 gm

Theoretical value = 0.300 gm

Percentage purity of Quinine sulphate $= \dfrac{0.376}{0.300} \times 100$

= 125.33%

RESULT

The percentage purity of given sample of Quinine sulphate tablet by fluorimetry was found to be 125.33% w/w.

EXPERIMENT 4.2B

Date ____________

ASSAY QUININE SULPHATE TABLET BY FLUORIMETRY
(Manual)

AIM

To perform the assay of quinine sulphate tablet by fluorimetry.

PROCEDURE

1. **Preparation of standard solution**
   (*a*) Weigh accurately 100 mg of Quinine sulphate powdered drug.
   (*b*) Dissolve in 100 ml of 0.1N H_2SO_4 (1 mg/ml).
   (*c*) Take 10 ml of above solution and dilute to 100 ml with 0.1N H_2SO_4 (100 μg/ml).
   (*d*) Again 10 ml of above solution dilute to 100 ml with 0.1N H_2SO_4 (10 μg/ml).
   (*e*) To get the resulting solution of 0.5, 1.0, 1.5, 2.0 and 2.5 μg/ml concentrations, take 0.5, 1.0, 1.5, 2.0 and 2.5 ml of above solutions respectively and dilute to 10 ml with 0.1N H_2SO_4.
2. **Preparation of sample (Quinine sulphate tablets)**
   (*a*) Weigh accurately 20 tablets and calculate the average weight.
   (*b*) Powder the tablets and weigh accurately the powdered quantity equivalent to 100 mg of quinine sulphate.
   (*c*) Dissolve in 75 ml of 0.1N H_2SO_4 by thorough mixing.
   (*d*) Make up the volume to 100 ml with 0.1N H_2SO_4 and filter.
   (*e*) Dilute 10 ml of above solution to 100 ml with 0.1N H_2SO_4.
   (*f*) Again take 10 ml of the solution and dilute to 100 ml with 0.1 N H_2SO_4.
   (*g*) To reach final concentration take 10 ml of the resulting solution and dilute to 100 ml to produce the concentration of 1 μg/ml.
3. Switch on the instrument. Set the excitation and emission filters at the wavelengths 365 and 459 respectively.
4. Set the fluorescence intensity to 0% by using 0.1N H_2SO_4 as blank and 100% by using highest concentration of the standard solution (2.5 μg/ml).
5. Repeat the same at least for two times more to minimize the instrumental error.
6. Measure the percentage fluorescence intensity of different standard and sample solutions.
7. Plot a graph between concentrations *vs.* F.I. and determine the concentration of unknown sample by extrapolating the found F.I.

OBSERVATIONS

1. Weight variation test

S. No.	Weight of tablet (gm)	Avg. wt. (gm)
1.		
2.		
3.		
4.		
5.		
6.		
7.		
8.		
9.		
10.		
11.		
12.		
13.		
14.		
15.		
16.		
17.		
18.		
19.		
20.		

2. Observation table

S. No.	Concentration	% F.I.
1.		
2		
3.		
4.		
5.		
6.		
7.	Sample	

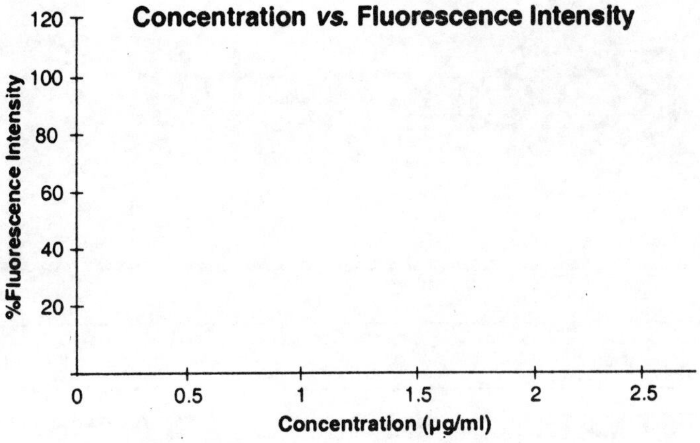

3. From graph, the concentration of Quinine sulphate drug = ________ μg/ml

CALCULATIONS

(*i*) Label claim of given tablet = 0.300 gm of Q.S.

(*ii*) Wt. of 20 tablets = ________ gm

(*iii*) Avg. wt. of each tablets = ________ gm

________ gm of powder contain = 0.300 gm of Q.S.

∴ *x* gm of powder = 0.100 gm of Q.S.

$$x = \frac{\_\_\_\_\_ \times \_\_\_\_\_}{\_\_\_\_\_}$$

∴ = ________ **gm**

CALCULATIONS

(*i*) From graph, initial quantity of drug that would be present in dilution

$$= \_\_\_\_\_ \times \_\_\_\_\_ \times \_\_\_\_\_ \times \_\_\_\_\_ \times \frac{100}{\_\_\_\_\_}$$

= ________ gm/100 ml

(*ii*) ∵ ________ gm of powder = 0.125 gm of Quinine sulphate

∴ ________ gm of powder will contain

= ________ × ________

= ________ gm of Quinine sulphate

Practical value = ________ gm

Theoretical value = 0.300 gm

Percentage purity of Quinine sulphate = ________ × 100

= ________%

RESULT

The percentage purity of given sample of Quinine sulphate tablet by fluorimetry was found to be ________% w/w.

Polarimetry

5

EXPERIMENT 5.1 A

Date ______________

ESTIMATION OF GLUCOSE BY POLARIMETRY

AIM

To find out the glucose (dextrose) content in a supplied sample by polarimetry.

PRINCIPLE

Polarimetric analysis is based on the optical activity of the substance, i.e. ability to rotate the plane-polarized light.

The rotatory power of a substance is expressed in terms of specific rotation. In case of solutions, specific rotation is

$$[\alpha]_{\lambda}^{t} = \frac{\alpha}{l.C}$$

α — Observed rotation of polarized beam at t°C

λ — Wavelength of light used

l — Length of liquid column in decimeter

C — Concentration of the solution in gm/ml

The accuracy and precision of optical rotation measurements can be increased if the following precautions are taken:

(*a*) The instrument must be in a good condition. The optical elements must be very clean and in exact alignment. The match point should be close to the normal zero mark.

(*b*) The light source should be properly aligned with respect to the optical bench. It should be supplemented by a filtering system capable of isolating the D line from sodium light.

(*c*) Specific attention should be paid to temperature control of the solution and of the polarimeter.

(*d*) Differences between the initial readings or between observed and corrected optical rotation, calculated, as either specific optical rotation or optical rotation, should not be more than one-fourth of the range specified in the monograph for the substance.

(*e*) Polarimeter tubes should be filled in such a way as to avoid air bubbles. Particular care is necessary for semi-micro or micro tubes.

(*f*) For tubes with removable end plates fitted with gaskets and caps, tighten the end-plates only enough to ensure a leak-proof seal between the end plate and the body of the tube.

(*g*) For substances with low rotatory power, the end-plates should be loosened and tightened again after each reading in the measurement of both the rotation and the zero point.

(*h*) Liquids and solutions of solids must be clear.

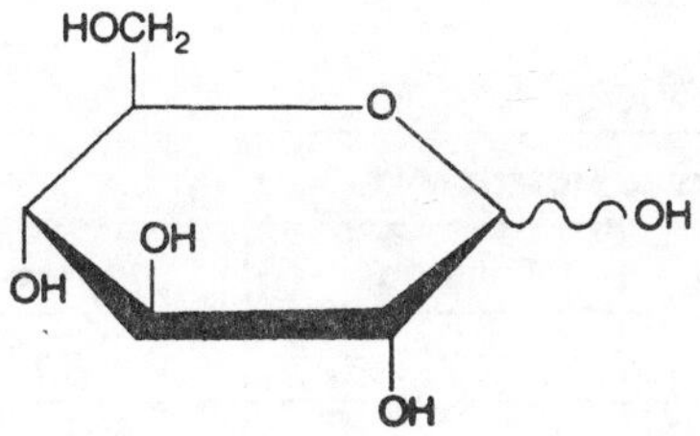

Mol. Formula: $C_6H_{12}O_6$ **Mol. Wt.:** 180.16 (anhydrous)

$C_6H_{12}O_6$, H_2O 198.17 (monohydrate)

Dextrose is D-(+)-glucopyranose or D-(+)-glucopyranose monohydrate.

Category: Nutrient; fluid replenisher.

Description: White crystalline powder.

Solubility: Freely soluble in *water*; sparingly soluble in *ethanol* (95%).

USES

Fluid replacement without significant electrolyte deficit; treatment of hypoglycemia.

PROCEDURE

1. Take 10 gm of glucose and transfer it into 100 ml volumetric flask.
2. Add 80 ml of distilled water to it and dissolve the solid by shaking.
3. Add 0.2 ml of 5 M ammonia, mix well and allow to stand for 30 minutes.
4. Make up the volume up to 100 ml with water.
5. Determine the zero point of the polarimeter.
6. Take five readings of the observed rotation of test solutions.
7. Take equal number of readings at the same time in the same tube with the solution for blank determination.
8. Take the average of both, i.e. test solution and solvent.
9. Find out the optical rotation.

OBSERVATIONS

1. Blank determination (for solvent)

S. No.	Observed Rotation		Observed Rotation Average	
	Degree	Division	Degree	Division
1.	350	3		
2.	351	2		
3.	354	3	352	3
4.	353	2		
5.	352	5		

$\because$ 9 divisions of fine scale measure = 1°

So 1 division of fine scale will measure ≡ 1°/9 = 0.11°

With blank the initial reading = 352° + (3 × 0.11°) = 352.33°

2. Final determination (for sample)

S. No.	Observed Rotation		Average	
	Degree	Division	Degree	Division
1.	360	5		
2.	362	4		
3.	362	3	360	4
4.	358	5		
5.	358	3		

With sample the final reading $\equiv 360 + (4 \times 0.11°) = 360.44$

3. Observed rotation (α)

$$= 360.44 - 352.33$$

$$= 8.11°$$

$$\text{Specific rotation } [\alpha]_\lambda' = \frac{\alpha}{l.C}$$

$$C = \frac{\alpha}{l \times [\alpha]_\lambda'} \quad \text{for glucose}$$

$$[\alpha]_\lambda' = 53°$$

$$l = 2 \text{ dm}$$

$$C = \frac{8.11}{2 \times 53}$$

$$= 0.0765 \text{ gm/ml}$$

$$\text{Sample solution will contain} = 0.0765 \times 100 \text{ gm/100 ml.}$$

$$= 7.65 \text{ gm/100 ml}$$

$$\text{\% Purity of sample} = \frac{\text{Practical value}}{\text{Theoretical value}} \times 100$$

$$= \frac{7.65}{10} \times 100 = 76.5\%$$

RESULT

The glucose content in the supplied sample by polarimetry was found to be 76.5%.

EXPERIMENT 5.1 B

Date ____________

ESTIMATION OF GLUCOSE BY POLARIMETRY

(Manual)

AIM

To find out the glucose (dextrose) content in a supplied sample by polarimetry.

PROCEDURE

1. Take 10 gm of glucose and transfer it into 100 ml volumetric flask.
2. Add 80 ml of distilled water to it and dissolve the solid by shaking.
3. Add 0.2 ml of 5 M ammonia, mix well and allow to stand for 30 minutes.
4. Make up the volume up to 100 ml with water.
5. Determine the zero point of the polarimeter.
6. Take five readings of the observed rotation of test solutions.
7. Take equal number of readings at the same time in the same tube with the solution for blank determination.
8. Take the average of both, i.e. test solution and solvent.
9. Find out the optical rotation.

OBSERVATIONS

1. Blank determination (for solvent)

S. No.	Observed Rotation		Observed Rotation (Average)	
	Degree	Division	Degree	Division
1.				
2.				
3.				
4.				
5.				

∵ 9 divisions of fine scale measure = 1°

So 1 division of fine scale will measure ≡ 1°/9 = 0.11°

With blank the initial reading = __________ + (3 × 0.11°)

= __________

2. Final determination (for sample)

S. No.	Observed Rotation		Observed Rotation (Average)	
	Degree	Division	Degree	Division
1.				
2.				
3.				
4.				
5.				

With sample the final reading = __________

3. Observed rotation (α) = __________ – __________

= __________

$$\text{Specific rotation } [\alpha]_\lambda^t = \frac{\alpha}{l.C}$$

$$C = \frac{\alpha}{l \times [\alpha]_\lambda^t} \text{ for glucose}$$

l = ___ _____ dm

C = __________ gm/ml

C = __________

Sample solution will contain = __________ gm/100 ml

__________ × 100 = __________ gm/100 ml

$$\text{Percentage purity of sample} = \frac{\text{Practical value}}{\text{Theoretical value}} \times 100$$

= __________ × 100

= __________%

RESULT

The glucose content in the supplied sample by polarimetry was found to be __________ %.

EXPERIMENT 5.2 A

Date ____________

ESTIMATION OF GLUCOSE BY POLARIMETRY

AIM

To find out the percentage of glucose content in the marketed product of glucose.

PRINCIPLE

Polarimetric analysis is based on the optical activity of the substance, i.e. ability to rotate the plane-polarized light. The rotatory power of a substance is expressed in terms of specific rotation. In case of solutions, specific rotation is

$$[\alpha]_\lambda^t = \frac{\alpha}{l.C}$$

α — Observed rotation of polarized beam at t° C

λ — Wavelength of light used

l — Length of liquid column in decimeter

C — Concentration of the solution in gm/ml

Polarimeter consists of

(*a*) A light source
(*b*) A polarizer for producing polarized radiation
(*c*) An analyzer, prism with a graduated scale to measure the amount of rotation
(*d*) Sample
(*e*) Detector tube

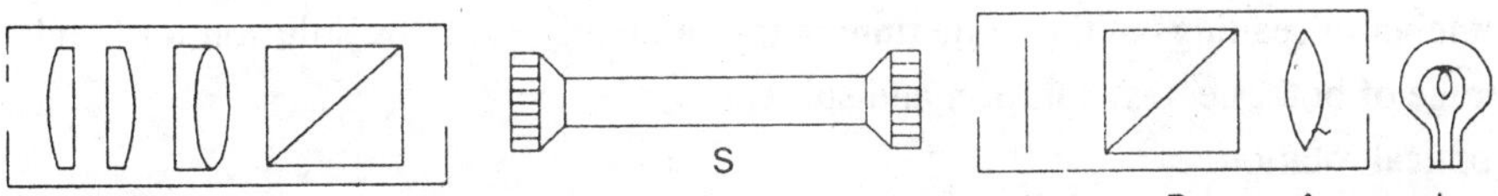

Polarimetry has widely been used in the quantitative analysis of optically active compounds, but its most important use is in the sugar industry.

The accuracy and precision of optical rotation measurements can be increased, if the following precautions are taken:

(*a*) The instrument must be in good condition. The optical elements must be very clean and in exact alignment. The match point should be closed to the normal zero mark.
(*b*) The light source should be properly aligned with respect to the optical bench. It should be supplemented by a filtering system capable of isolating the D line from sodium light.
(*c*) Specific attention should be paid to temperature control of the solution and of the polarimeter.
(*d*) Differences between the initial readings or between observed and corrected optical rotation, calculated, as either specific optical rotation or optical rotation, should not be more than one-fourth of the range specified in the monograph for the substance.
(*e*) Polarimeter tubes should be filled in such a way as to avoid air bubbles. Particular care is necessary for semi-micro or micro tubes.
(*f*) For tubes with removable end-plates fitted with gaskets and caps, tighten the end-plates only enough to ensure a leak-proof seal between the end-plate and the body of the tube.
(*g*) For substances with low rotatory power, the end-plates should be loosened and tightened again after each reading, in the measurement of both the rotation and the zero point.

(*h*) Liquids and solutions of solids must be clear.

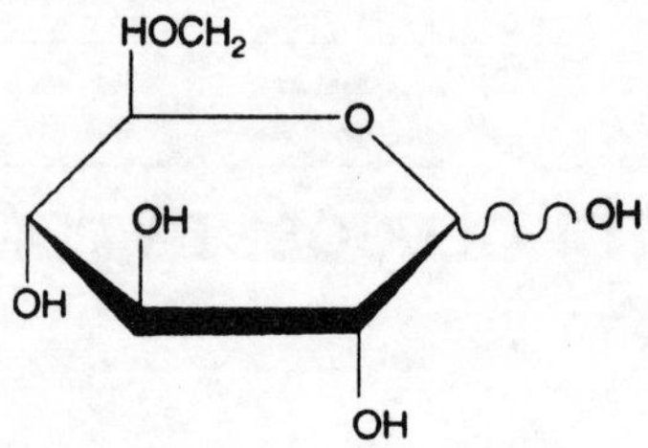

Mol. Formula: $C_6H_{12}O_6$ (anhydrous) **Mol. Wt.:** 180.16

$C_6H_{12}O_6$, H_2O (monohydrate) 198.17

Dextrose is D-(+)-glucopyranose or D-(+)-glucopyranose monohydrate.

Category: Nutrient; fluid replenisher.

Description: White crystalline powder.

Solubility: Freely soluble in water; sparingly soluble in ethanol (95%).

USES

Fluid replacement without significant electrolyte deficit; treatment of hypoglycemia.

PROCEDURE

1. Take 10 gm of glucose and transfer it into 100 ml volumetric flask.
2. Add 80 ml of distilled water to it and dissolve the solid by shaking.
3. Add 0.2 ml of 5 M ammonia, mix well and allow to stand for 30 minutes.
4. Make up the volume up to 100 ml with water.
5. Determine the zero point of the polarimeter.
6. Take five readings of the observed rotation of test solutions.
7. Take equal number of readings at the same time in the same tube with the solution for blank determination.
8. Take the average of both, i.e. test solution and solvent.
9. Find out the optical rotation.

OBSERVATIONS

1. Label claim

Each 100 gm of powder contains = 99.4 gm of Dextrose

So each 10 gm of powder will contain = 9.94 gm of Dextrose

∴ Concentration of sample solution = 9.94 gm/100 ml

2. Blank determination (solvent)

S. No.	Observed Rotation		Observed Rotation (Average)	
	Degree	Division	Degree	Division
1.	300	3		
2.	351	2		
3.	354	3	352	3
4.	353	2		
5.	352	5		

$\because$ 9 divisions of fine scale measure $= 1°$

So 1 division of fine scale will measure $\equiv 1°/9 = 0.11°$

With blank the initial reading $= 352° + (3 \times 0.11°) = 352.33°$

3. Final determination (sample)

S. No.	Observed Rotation		Observed Rotation (Average)	
	Degree	Division	Degree	Division
1.	360	5		
2.	362	4		
3.	362	3	360	4
4.	358	5		
5.	358	3		

With sample the final reading $\equiv 360 + (4 \times 0.11°) = 360.44$

4. Observed rotation (α) $= 360.44 - 352.33 = 8.11°$

$$\text{Specific rotation } [\alpha]_{\lambda}^{t} = \frac{\alpha}{l.C}$$

$$C = \frac{\alpha}{l \times [\alpha]_{\lambda}^{t}} \qquad \text{For glucose}$$

$$[\alpha]_{\lambda}^{t} = 53°$$

$$l = 2 \text{ dm}$$

$$C = \frac{8.11}{2 \times 53}$$

$$= 0.0765 \text{ gm/ml}$$

$$= 0.0765 \times 100 \text{ gm/100 ml}$$

$$= 0.765 \text{ gm/100 ml}$$

$$\text{Purity of sample} = \frac{7.65}{9.94} \times 100 = 76.96\%$$

RESULT

The glucose content in the marketed product of glucose by polarimetry was found to be 76.96%.

EXPERIMENT 5.2B

Date ____________

ESTIMATION OF GLUCOSE BY POLARIMETRY
(Manual)

AIM

To find out the percentage of glucose content in the marketed product of glucose.

PROCEDURE

1. Take 10 gm of glucose and transfer it into 100 ml volumetric flask.
2. Add 80 ml of distilled water to it and dissolve the solid by shaking.
3. Add 0.2 ml of 5 M ammonia, mix well and allow to stand for 30 minutes.
4. Make up the volume up to 100 ml with water.
5. Determine the zero point of the polarimeter.
6. Take five readings of the observed rotation of test solutions.
7. Take equal number of readings at the same time in the same tube with the solution for blank determination.
8. Take the average of both, i.e. test solution and solvent.
9. Find out the optical rotation.

OBSERVATIONS

1. Label claim

Each 100 gm of powder contains = __________ gm of Dextrose

So each 10 gm of powder will contain = __________ gm of Dextrose

∴ Concentration of sample solution = __________ gm/100 ml

2. Blank determination (solvent)

S. No.	Observed Rotation		Observed Rotation (Average)	
	Degree	Division	Degree	Division
1.				
2.				
3.				
4.				
5.				

∵ 9 divisions of fine scale measure = 1°

So 1 division of fine scale will measure ≡ 1°/9 = 0.11°

With blank the initial reading = __________°

3. Final determination (sample)

S. No.	Observed Rotation		Observed Rotation (Average)	
	Degree	Division	Degree	Division
1.				
2.				
3.				
4.				
5.				

With sample the final reading = __________

4. Observed rotation (α) = __________

$$\text{Specific rotation } [\alpha]_{\lambda}^{t} = \frac{\alpha}{l.C}$$

$$C = \frac{\alpha}{l \times [\alpha]_{\lambda}^{t}} \quad \text{For glucose}$$

$[\alpha]_{\lambda}^{t}$ = __________

l = __________ dm

C = __________

C = __________ gm/ml

= __________ × 100

Purity of sample = __________%

RESULT

The glucose content in the marketed product of glucose by polarimetry was found to be __________%.

EXPERIMENT 5.3 A

Date ____________

ESTIMATION OF GLUCOSE BY POLARIMETRY

AIM

To find out the glucose content in the marketed product of dextrose injection I.P.

PRINCIPLE

Polarimetric analysis is based on the optical activity of the substance i.e. ability to rotate the plane-polarized light.

The rotatory power of a substance is expressed in terms of specific rotation. In case of solutions, specific rotation is

$$[\alpha]_{\lambda}^{t} = \frac{\alpha}{l.C}$$

α — Observed rotation of polarized beam at $t°$ C
λ — Wavelength of light used
l — Length of liquid column in decimeter.
C — Concentration of the solution in gm/ml.

PROCEDURE

1. Take an accurately measured volume of glucose IV infusion equivalent to 4 gm of glucose.
2. Add 80 ml of distilled water to it and dissolve the solid by shaking.
3. Add 0.2 ml of 5 M ammonia, mix well and allow to stand for 30 minutes.
4. Make up the volume up to 100 ml with water.
5. Determine the zero point of the polarimeter.
6. Take five readings of the observed rotation of test solutions.
7. Take equal number of readings at the same time in the same tube with the solution for blank determination.
8. Take the average of both, i.e. test solution and solvent.
9. Find out the optical rotation.

OBSERVATIONS

1. Blank determination (solvent)

S. No.	Observed Rotation		Observed Rotation (Average)	
	Degree	Division	Degree	Division
1.	350	3		
2.	351	2		
3.	354	3	352	3
4.	353	2		
5.	352	5		

$\because$ 9 divisions of fine scale measure = 1°

So 1 division of fine scale will measure $\equiv$ 1°/9 = 0.11°

With blank the initial reading = 352° + (3 × 0.11°) = 352.33°

2. Final determination (sample)

S. No.	Observed Rotation		Observed Rotation (Average)	
	Degree	Division	Degree	Division
1.	360	5		
2.	362	4		
3.	362	3	360	4
4.	358	5		
5.	358	3		

With sample the final reading $\equiv$ 360 + (4 × 0.11°) = 360.44

3. Observed rotation (α) = 360.44 – 352.33 = 8.11°

Observed rotation (α) × 0.9447 = Wt. in gm of glucose in the volume taken

100 ml of sample solution will contain = 8.11 × 0.9447 gm of glucose

= 7.66 gm/100 ml

$$\% \text{ Purity of sample} = \frac{\text{Practical value}}{\text{Theoretical value}} \times 100$$

$$= \frac{7.66}{10} \times 100 = 76.6\%$$

RESULT

The glucose content in the marketed product of Dextrose injection I.P. by polarimetry was found to be 76.6%.

EXPERIMENT 5.3B

Date ____________

ESTIMATION OF GLUCOSE BY POLARIMETRY
(Manual)

AIM

To find out the glucose content in the marketed product of dextrose injection I.P.

PROCEDURE

1. Take an accurately measured volume of glucose IV infusion equivalent to 4 gm of glucose.
2. Add 80 ml of distilled water to it and dissolve the solid by shaking.
3. Add 0.2 ml of 5 M ammonia, mix well and allow to stand for 30 minutes.
4. Make up the volume up to 100 ml with water.
5. Determine the zero point of the polarimeter.
6. Take five readings of the observed rotation of test solutions.
7. Take equal number of readings at the same time in the same tube with the solution for blank determination.
8. Take the average of both, i.e. test solution and solvent.
9. Find out the optical rotation.

OBSERVATIONS

1. Blank determination (solvent)

S. No.	Observed Rotation		Observed Rotation (Average)	
	Degree	Division	Degree	Division
1.				
2.				
3.				
4.				
5.				

∵ 9 divisions of fine scale measure = 1°

So 1 division of fine scale will measure ≡ 1°/9 = 0.11°

With blank the initial reading = __________°

2. Final determination (sample)

S. No.	Observed Rotation		Observed Rotation (Average)	
	Degree	Division	Degree	Division
1.				
2.				
3.				
4.				
5.				

With sample the final reading = __________

3. Observed rotation (α) = __________°

Observed rotation (α) × __________ = Wt. in gm of glucose in the volume taken

100 ml of sample solution will contain = __________ gm/100 ml

$$\% \text{ purity of sample} = \frac{\text{Practical value}}{\text{Theoretical value}} \times 100$$

= __________

= __________ %

RESULT

The glucose content in the marketed product of Dextrose injection I.P. by polarimetry was found to be _______ %.

EXPERIMENT 5.4 A

Date ____________

ESTIMATION OF GLUCOSE BY POLARIMETRY

AIM

To find out the percentage of glucose content in the marketed product of oral rehydration salt (ORS).

THEORY

If the fluid loss is mild (5–7%) or moderate (7.5–10%), oral rehydration therapy can be instituted from very beginning.

Rationale of ORS composition

Oral dehydration is possible if glucose is added with salt. This is glucose facilitated Na^+ absorption. Intestinal fluid locks glucose, so it can not be absorbed. ORS should be isotonic and the molar ratio of glucose should be somewhat higher than Na^+. Excess glucose will be utilized in absorbing Na^+ present in the intestinal secretions in addition to that present in ORS itself. Enough K^+ and HCO_3^- should be provided to make up the losses in stool.

The WHO has recommended a universal formula:

$$\left.\begin{aligned} NaCl &= 3.5\text{ g} \\ KCl &= 1.5\text{ g} \\ \text{Sodium citrate} &= 2.9\text{ g} \\ \text{Glucose} &= 2.0\text{ g} \end{aligned}\right\}\text{ to be dissolved in 1 litre of water}$$

PROCEDURE

1. Take about 10 gm of glucose sample in 100 ml volumetric flask and then dissolve in 75 ml of water.
2. Add 0.2 ml of ammonia and make up the volume to 100 ml with water.
3. Filter the solution to remove turbidity.
4. Firstly, fill the blank solution in sample tube and set the zero reading of the polarimeter.
5. Rinse the sample tube twice with the sample and then finally observe the angle of rotation of the sample.
6. Calculate the optical rotation of given substance.

PRECAUTION

1. Sample solution must be transparent.
2. Sample tube should not contain any air bubble in the track of liquid sample.
3. The experiment should not be started until the light of polarimeter becomes yellow from pink.

OBSERVATIONS AND CALCULATIONS

1. Initial reading (zero reading) determined for blank is 352.33° (initial).
2. Determination of sample reading, i.e. final reading.
   (*a*) On placement of sample solution in sample tube:

S. No.	Observation	Inference
1.	Field is half bright and half dark	Solution contain optically active substance.
2.	Right hand side half field is bright	Optically active substance is dextrorotatory.

(*b*) Determination of optical rotation with sample solution field becomes uniform at

$$= 359° + 3 \text{ div.} = 359.33°$$

$$\text{Observed rotation} = \text{final reading} - \text{initial reading}$$

$$= 359.33° - 352.33 = 7°$$

$$\text{Specific rotation } [\alpha] = \frac{\alpha}{l.C.}$$

$$C = \frac{\alpha}{\lambda\,[\alpha]_\lambda^t}$$

$$= \frac{7}{2 \times 53} = 0.0660 \text{ gm/ml}$$

So 100 ml sample solution will contain

$$= 6.60 \text{ gm} = 6.6\%$$

Theoretical concentration:

Weight of sample = 10 gm

10 gm sample shows = 6.6 gm dextrose

So 100 gm sample shows = 66.0%

% purity of supplied compound = 66.0%

RESULT

The % of glucose content found is 66.0%, label claims 50%. So it does not comply with I.P. limits.

EXPERIMENT 5.4 B

Date ______________

ESTIMATION OF GLUCOSE BY POLARIMETRY
(Manual)

AIM

To find out the percentage of glucose content in the marketed product of oral rehydration salt (ORS).

PROCEDURE

1. Take about 10 gm of glucose sample in 100 ml volumetric flask and then dissolve in 75 ml of water.
2. Add 0.2 ml of ammonia and make up the volume to 100 ml with water.
3. Filter the solution to remove turbidity.
4. Firstly, fill the blank solution in sample tube and set the zero reading of the polarimeter.
5. Rinse the sample tube twice with the sample and then finally observe the angle of rotation of the sample.
6. Calculate the optical rotation of given substance.

PRECAUTION

1. Sample solution must be transparent.
2. Sample tube should not contain any air bubble in the track of liquid sample.
3. Experiment should not be started until the light of polarimeter becomes yellow from pink.

OBSERVATIONS AND CALCULATIONS

1. Initial reading (zero reading) determined for blank is ____________° (initial).
2. Determination of sample reading, i.e. final reading.

(*a*) On placement of sample solution in sample tube

S. No.	Observation	Inference
1.	Field is half bright and half dark	Solution contain optically active substance.
2.	Right hand side half field is bright	Optically active substance is dextrorotatory.

(*b*) Determination of optical rotation with sample solution, field becomes uniform at

= ____________°

Observed rotation = final reading – initial reading

$$\text{Specific rotation } [\alpha] = \frac{\alpha}{l.C}$$

$$C = \frac{\alpha}{\lambda[\alpha]^{t}_{\lambda}} = \text{\_\_\_\_\_\_\_\_\_\_ gm/ml}$$

So 100 ml sample solution will contain

= ____________ gm

= ____________ %

Theoretical concentration

Weight of sample = 10 gm

10 gm sample shows = __________ gm dextrose

So 100 gm sample shows = __________ %

Percentage purity of supplied compound = __________ %

RESULT

The percentage of glucose content found is __________%, label claims __________ %.

Conductometry

6

EXPERIMENT 6.1 A

Date ______________

CONDUCTOMETRIC TITRATION OF ACID

AIM

To determine the end-point and normality of given acid by conductometric titration.

PRINCIPLE

Conductometry is the determination of conductance due to presence of ions in the solutions by conductometer. The conductivity **(c)** depends upon the mobility or migration of the cations ($H^{\oplus}$, $Na^{\oplus}$, $K^{\oplus}$ and $NH_4^{\oplus}$ etc.) and anions (like OH^-, Cl^-, I^-, Br^-, SO_4^{-2} and CO_3^{-2} etc.) present in the solutions towards their respective electrodes. Conductivity is inversely proportional to resistance **(R),** depends upon the concentration of ions present in solution, charge of ions, size of ions and temperature etc.

$$R_{(\text{ohm})} = \frac{V}{I}$$

Where,

V = Potential difference

I = Current flow

R = Resistance

$$\underset{(\text{mho or ohm}^{-1})}{\text{Conductance}} = \frac{1}{\text{Resistance } (R)}$$

The principle behind this experiment is when HCl is taken in beaker, the initial conductivity is high because the strong acid completely dissociates into $H^{\oplus}$ and as NaOH is added, the OH^- of NaOH reacts with $H^{\oplus}$ to produce water. As a result conductivity gradually decreases after every addition.

At the end-point, when all the $H^{\oplus}$ of acid (HCl) reacts with OH^- to produce water, now the addition of NaOH further increases the conductance of OH^- and a "X" shaped graph is obtained.

Ions	Ionic conductivity ($\lambda \times 10^{-4}$)
$H^{\oplus}$	350
OH^-	199
Cl^-	76
$Na^{\oplus}$	50
CH_3COO^-	41

PROCEDURE

1. Switch on the conductometer and allow to stabilize for 30 minutes.
2. Take 50 ml of 0.1N HCl in a beaker and 1N NaOH solution in the burette.
3. Insert the platinum electrodes in the beaker.
4. Determine the initial conductance of acid.
5. Titrate the acid with 1N NaOH solution by adding 1 ml at a time and note the conductivity of the solution.
6. Take several readings before and after the approximate end-point.
7. Plot a graph between conductance observed and volume of the titrant added.
8. Determine the end-point from graph.
9. Calculate the normality of acid.

OBSERVATION TABLE

S. No.	Vol. of 1 N NaOH added (ml)	Conductivity (mho)
1.	0	4.85
2.	1	4.7
3.	2	4.1
4.	3	3.45
5.	4	2.9
6.	5	2.3
7.	6	1.8
8.	7	1.2
9.	8	1.5
10.	9	1.8
11.	10	2.15
12.	11	2.45
13.	12	2.75

NaOH *vs.* Conductivity

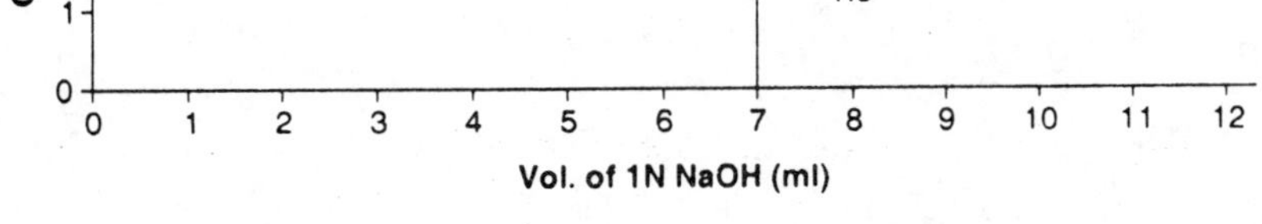

CALCULATION

$$N_1 V_1 = N_2 V_2$$

Where

N_1 = Normality of NaOH = 1 N

N_2 = Normality of acid (HCl) = ?

V_1 = Volume of NaOH consumed = 7 ml (from graph)

V_2 = Volume of acid taken = 50 ml

$$1 \times 7 = N_2 \times 50$$

$$N_2 = 0.14 \text{ N}$$

RESULT

The normality of the given acid, Hydrochloric acid was found to be **0.14 N.**

EXPERIMENT 6.1 B

Date ____________

CONDUCTOMETRIC TITRATION OF ACID

(Manual)

AIM

To determine the end-point and normality of given acid by conductometric titration.

PROCEDURE

1. Switch on the conductometer and allow to stabilize for 30 minutes.
2. Take 50 ml of 0.1N HCl in a beaker and 1N NaOH solution in the burette.
3. Insert the platinum electrodes in the beaker.
4. Determine the initial conductance of acid.
5. Titrate the acid with 1N NaOH solution by adding 1 ml at a time and note the conductivity of the solution.
6. Take several readings before and after the approximate end-point.
7. Plot a graph between conductance observed and volume of the titrant added.
8. Determine the end-point from graph.
9. Calculate the normality of acid.

OBSERVATION TABLE

S. No.	Vol. of 1 N NaOH added (ml)	Conductivity (mho)
1.		
2.		
3.		
4.		
5.		
6.		
7.		
8.		
9.		
10.		
11.		
12.		
13.		

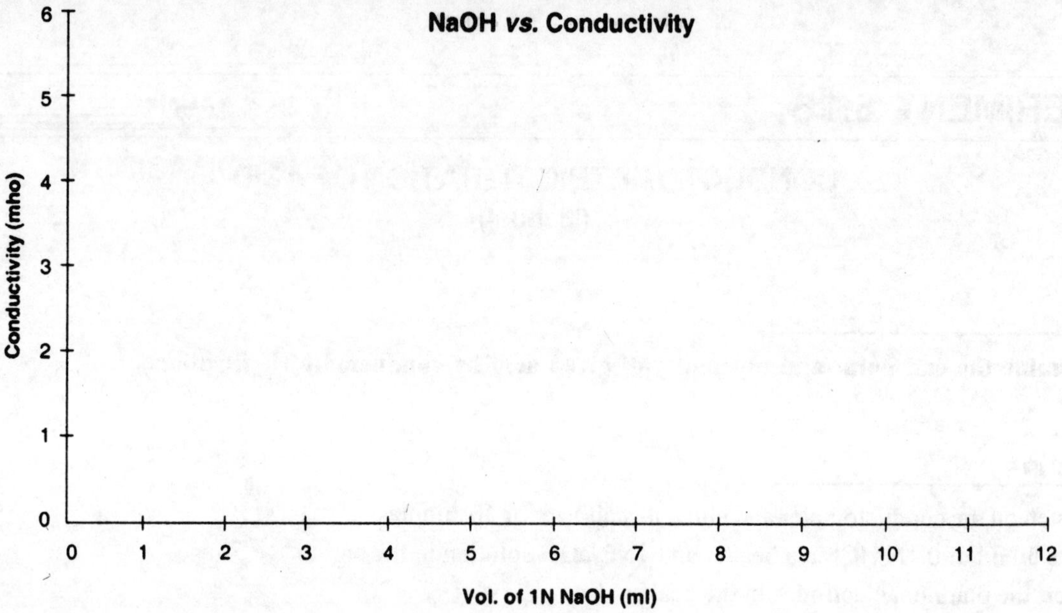

CALCULATION

$$N_1 V_1 = N_2 V_2$$

Where

N_1 = Normality of NaOH = 1 N

N_2 = Normality of acid (HCl) = ?

V_1 = Volume of NaOH consumed = __________ ml (from graph)

V_2 = Volume of acid taken = 50 ml

N_2 = __________N

RESULT

The normality of the given acid, Hydrochloric acid was found to be __________ N.

EXPERIMENT 6.2A

Date ____________

CONDUCTOMETRIC TITRATION OF MIXTURE OF ACIDS

AIM

To carry out the conductometric titration of mixture of acids [0.1N HCl + 0.1N CH_3COOH] *vs.* strong base (1N NaOH).

PRINCIPLE

Conductometry is the determination of conductance due to presence of ions in the solutions by conductometer. The conductivity C depends upon the mobility or migration of the cations ($H^{\oplus}$, $Na^{\oplus}$, $K^{\oplus}$ and $NH_4^{\oplus}$ etc.) and anions (like OH^-, Cl^-, I^-, Br^-, SO_4^{-2} and CO_3^{-2} etc.) present in the solutions towards their respective electrodes. Conductivity is inversely proportional to resistance R, depends upon the concentration of ions present in solution, charge of ions, size of ions and temperature etc.

$$R\,(\text{ohm}) = \frac{V}{I}$$

Where:

V = Potential difference

I = Current flow

R = Resistance

$$\underset{(\text{mho or ohm}^{-1})}{\text{Conductance}} = \frac{1}{\text{Resistance } (R)}$$

The principle behind the experiment is when HCl is taken in beaker, the initial conductivity is high because the strong acid completely dissociates into $H^{\oplus}$ and as NaOH is added, the OH^- of NaOH reacts with $H^{\oplus}$ to produce water. As a result conductivity gradually decreases after every addition.

At the end-point when all the $H^{\oplus}$ of acid (HCl) reacts with OH^- to produce water, now the addition of NaOH further increases the conductance of OH^-.

In conductometric titration of mixture of acids (0.1N HCl + 0.1N CH_3COOH), when a solution of NaOH is added, the OH^- reacts with $H^{\oplus}$ of HCl to produce water and conductivity decreases, at the same time $Na^{\oplus}$ reacts with CH_3COOH to form CH_3COONa salt and as a result conductivity slightly rises due to $H^{\oplus}$ of CH_3COOH. It should be noted that the CH_3COOH is a weak acid and its initial conductivity is low.

After the end-point, further the addition of NaOH causes increase in conductivity due to OH^- and a "*V*" shaped graph is obtained.

Ions	Ionic conductivity ($\lambda \times 10^{-4}$)
$H^{\oplus}$	350
OH^-	199
Cl^-	76
$Na^{\oplus}$	50
CH_3COO^-	41

PROCEDURE

1. Switch on the conductometer and allow to stabilize for 30 minutes.
2. Take 75 ml of 0.1N HCl and 25 ml of 0.1N CH_3COOH in a beaker and NaOH in the burette.
3. Insert the platinum electrodes in the beaker.
4. Determine the initial conductance of acid mixture.
5. Titrate the acid mixture with 1N NaOH solution by adding 1 ml at a time and note the conductivity of the solution.
6. Take several readings before and after the approximate end-point.
7. Plot a graph between conductance observed and volume of the titrant added.
8. Determine the end-point from graph.
9. Calculate the normality of acids.

OBSERVATION TABLE

S. No.	Vol. of 1 N NaOH added (ml)	Conductivity (mho)
1.	0	2.6
2.	1	2.8
3.	2	2.7
4.	3	2.4
5.	4	2.2
6.	5	1.9
7.	6	1.6
8.	7	1.4
9.	8	0.9
10.	9	0.9
11.	10	0.9
12.	11	1.0
13.	12	1.1
14.	13	1.2
15.	14	1.3
16.	15	1.4
17.	16	1.6
18.	17	1.8
19.	18	1.9
20.	19	2.0
21.	20	2.1
22.	21	2.1

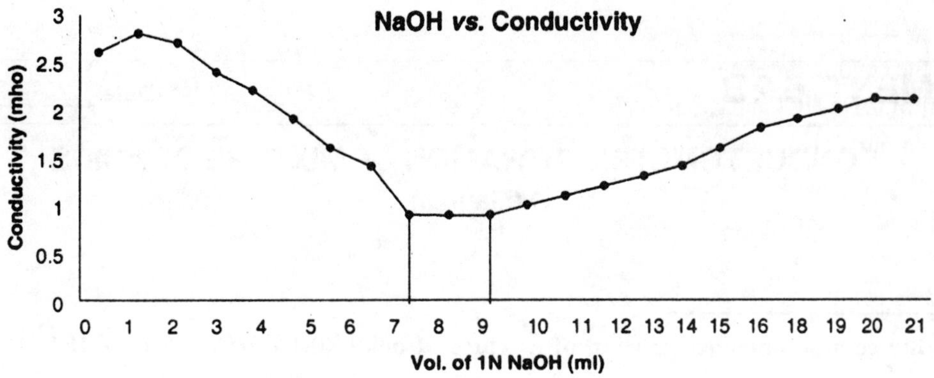

Form Graph

Volume of NaOH consumed for HCl = 8 ml

Volume of NaOH consumed for CH_3COOH = 10 – 8 = 2 ml

CALCULATION

1. For HCl

$$N_1 V_1 = N_2 V_2$$

N_1 = Normality of NaOH = 1 N

V_1 = Volume of NaOH consumed = 8 ml

N_2 = Normality of HCl = ?

V_2 = Volume of HCl taken = 75 ml

$$N_2 = \frac{8 \times 1}{75} = 0.1066 \text{ N}$$

2. For CH_3COOH

$$N_3 V_3 = N_4 V_4$$

N_3 = Normality of NaOH = 1 N

V_3 = Volume of NaOH consumed = 10 – 8 = 2 ml

N_4 = Normality of CH_3COOH = ?

V_4 = Volume of CH_3COOH taken = 25 ml

$$N_4 = \frac{2}{25} = 0.08 \text{ N}$$

RESULT

The normality of acids by conductometric titration were found to be

HCl = 0.1066 N

CH_3COOH = 0.08 N

EXPERIMENT 6.2B

Date ________________

CONDUCTOMETRIC TITRATION OF MIXTURE OF ACIDS (Manual)

AIM

To carry out the conductometric titration of mixture of acids [0.1N HCl + 0.1N CH_3COOH] *vs.* strong base (1N NaOH).

PROCEDURE

1. Switch on the conductometer and allow to stabilize for 30 minutes.
2. Take 75 ml of 0.1N HCl and 25 ml of 0.1N CH_3COOH in a beaker and NaOH in the burette.
3. Insert the platinum electrodes in the beaker.
4. Determine the initial conductance of acid mixture.
5. Titrate the acid mixture with 1N NaOH solution by adding 1 ml at a time and note the conductivity of the solution.
6. Take several readings before and after the approximate end-point.
7. Plot a graph between conductance observed and volume of the titrant added.
8. Determine the end-point from graph.
9. Calculate the normality of acids.

OBSERVATION TABLE

S. No.	Vol. of 1 N NaOH added (ml)	Conductivity(μ mho)
1.		
2.		
3.		
4.		
5.		
6.		
7.		
8.		
9.		
10.		
11.		
12.		
13.		
14.		
15.		

(*Contd.*)

S. No.	Vol. of 1 N NaOH added (ml)	Conductivity(μ mho)
16.		
17.		
18.		
19.		
20.		
21.		
22.		

NaOH *vs.* Conductivity

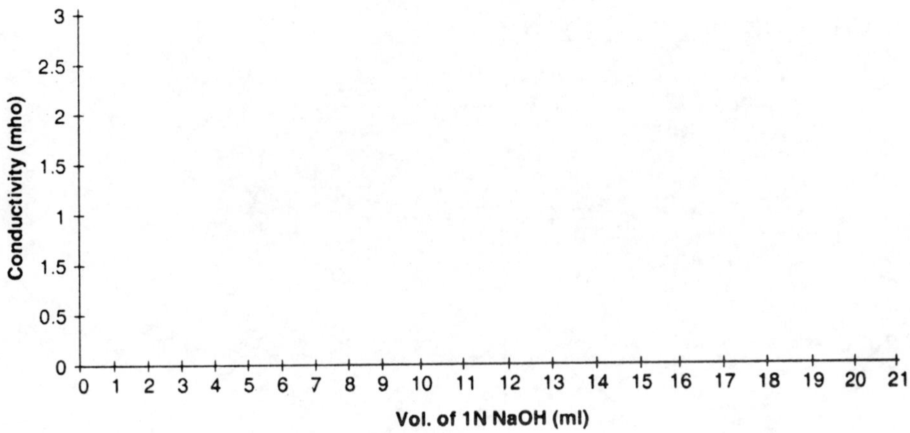

From Graph

Volume of NaOH consumed for HCl = __________ ml

Volume of NaOH consumed for CH_3COOH = __________ ml

CALCULATION

1. For HCl

$$N_1 V_1 = N_2 V_2$$

N_1 = Normality of NaOH = 1 N

V_1 = Volume of NaOH consumed = __________ ml

N_2 = Normality of HCl = ?

V_2 = Volume of HCl taken = __________ ml

$$N_2 = \frac{\_\_\_\_ \times \_\_\_\_}{\_\_\_\_}$$

$$= \_\_\_\_\_\_\_\_ \text{ N}$$

2. For CH_3COOH

$N_3 V_3 = N_4 V_4$

N_3 = Normality of NaOH = 1 N

V_3 = Volume of NaOH consumed = __________ ml

N_4 = Normality of CH_3COOH = ?

V_4 = Volume of CH_3COOH taken = __________ ml

N_4 = $\frac{\_\_\_\_\_\_\_\_}{\_\_\_\_\_}$ = ________ N

RESULT

The normality of acids by conductometric titration were found to be

HCl = __________ N

CH_3COOH = __________ N

Refractometry

7

EXPERIMENT 7.1 A

Date ______________

DETERMINATION OF R.I. OF LIQUIDS BY ABBES REFRACTOMETER

AIM

To find out the refractive indices of different liquids (benzene, glycerin and water) by abbes refractometer.

THEORY

When a beam of light is allowed to pass from rare (air) into a denser medium such as liquid, the beam suffers refraction. According to Snell's law, the ratio of the sine of the angle of incidence and refraction is constant and is called as the refractive index of the liquid.

$$n = \frac{\sin i}{\sin r}$$

i = angle of incidence

r = angle of refraction

n is refractive index of the liquid.

The refractive index is a physical property of the liquids used to identify them.

Abbe's Refractometer

It essentially consists of a two glass prism A and B. The surface of B prism is polished, while that of A is finely ground. The two prisms are enclosed in metal casing hinged at H. The two prisms can be rotated about a horizontal axis immediately beneath a telescope T and they can be held in contact with the help of a clamp C. An arm R which is attached with the metal case carrying the prisms move along a graduated scale, the reading of which gives directly the refractive index of the liquid under examination.

Mechanism

The beam of light passes from a suitable source is reflected by the mirror M, passes through the lower prism A and illuminates the upper surface PR. A drop of liquid under examination is placed upon the surface of A. On clamping the prism A and B, a film of the liquid spreads between them. The light is refracted by mirror M is scattered into the liquid film at different angle of incidence. A particular ray going along the grazing incidence will pass through the prism B at an angle i which is equal to the critical angle.

$$\sin i = (n/N)$$

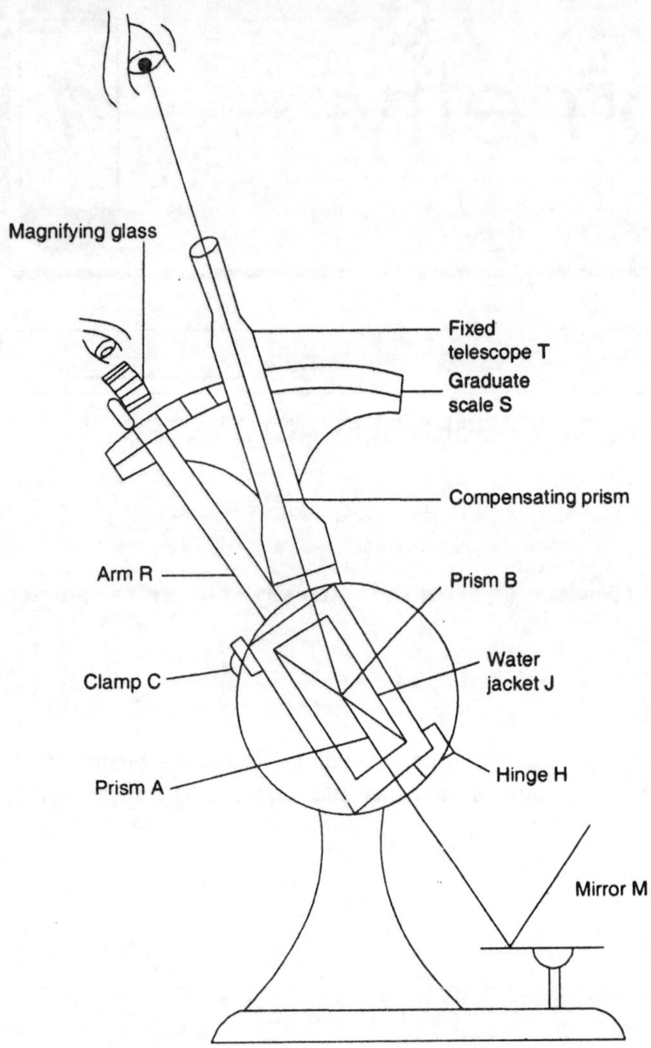

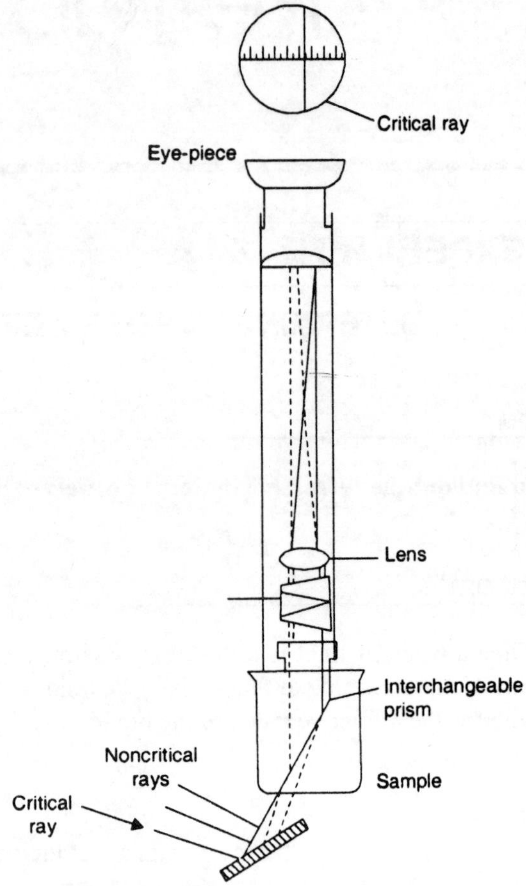

PROCEDURE

1. Clean the surfaces of the prism with dry cotton and then clean them with distilled water.
2. Again clean with acetone and finally wipe the surface with dry cotton.
3. Place a drop of pure benzene on the surface.
4. Now clamp the prism A and B in order to make a film between them.
5. View through the telescope in such a way that the field of view should be equally dividing into light and dark portion.
6. It should be noted that the bright portion should coincide with the cross wire of the telescope.
7. Note the reading and least-count on the scale.
8. Calćulate the refractive index of the benzene
9. Adopt the same procedure for water and glycerin also.

OBSERVATIONS

1. Distilled water

$$\text{R.I.} = 1.32 + 9 \text{ divisions}$$

$$\text{Least-count: } 10 \text{ divisions} = 0.01 \text{ R.I.}$$

$$9 \text{ divisions} = \frac{0.01 \times 9}{10} = 0.009$$

$$\text{R.I.} = 1.32 + 0.009 = 1.329$$

2. Glycerin

$$\text{R.I.} = 1.50 + (10 \text{ divisions})$$

$$= 1.50 + (0.001 \times 10)$$

$$= 1.510$$

3. Benzene

$$\text{R.I.} = 1.53 + (9 \times 0.001)$$

$$= 1.539$$

RESULTS

The observed R.I. by Abbe's refractometer of samples are:

Distilled water = 1.329

Glycerin = 1.510

Benzene = 1.539

EXPERIMENT 7.1 B

Date ____________

DETERMINATION OF R.I. OF LIQUIDS BY ABBES REFRACTOMETER (Manual)

AIM

To find out the refractive indices of different liquids (benzene, glycerin and water) by abbes refractometer.

PROCEDURE

1. Clean the surfaces of the prism with dry cotton and then clean them with distilled water.
2. Again clean with acetone and finally wipe the surface with dry cotton.
3. Place a drop of pure benzene on the surface.
4. Now clamp the prism A and B in order to make a film between them.
5. View through the telescope in such a way that the field of view should be equally dividing into light and dark portion.
6. It should be noted that the bright portion should coincide with the cross wire of the telescope.
7. Note the reading and least-count on the scale.
8. Calculate the refractive index of the benzene.
9. Adopt the same procedure for water and glycerin also.

OBSERVATIONS

1. Distilled water

R.I. = __________ + (__________ division)

Least-count: 10 divisions = 0.01 R.I.

R.I. = __________

2. Glycerin

R.I. = __________ + (__________ division)

= __________

3. Benzene

R.I. = __________

RESULTS

The observed R.I. by Abbe's refractometer of samples are:

Distilled water = __________

Glycerin = __________

Benzene = __________

EXPERIMENT 7.2 A

Date ______

MOLAR REFRACTION OF BENZENE BY ABBE'S REFRACTOMETER

AIM

To find out the molar refraction of benzene by abbe's refractometer and also confirm the structure of benzene.

PRINCIPLE

When the beam of light is allowed to pass from rare (air) into denser medium such as liquid, the beam suffers refraction. According to Snell's law, the ratio of the sine of the angle of incidence and refraction is constant and is called as the refractive index of the liquid.

$$n = \frac{\sin i}{\sin r}$$

i = angle of incidence

r = angle of refraction

n is refractive index of the liquid.

The R.I. is a physical property of the liquids used to identify them.

Specific refraction may be defined by the equation:

$$R = \frac{n^2 - 1}{n^2 + 2} \times \frac{1}{d}$$

Where

n = R.I. of liquid

d = density of liquid

R = specific rotation

The advantage of Specific Rotation is that, it is independent of temperature. Since the change in R.I. is compensated by the change in density of the liquid. If the specific rotation is multiplied by molecular weight of the substance, the product is called as Molar Refractivity.

$$\text{M.R.} = [R] = \frac{n^2 - 1}{n^2 + 2} \times \frac{1}{d} \times M$$

Where M = Molecular weight of the substance

Applications of molar refraction

1. The composition of binary liquid or gaseous mixtures can be easily and conveniently determined by refractive index.
2. The determination of concentration of aqueous sugar solution is the most important quantitative application of molar refraction.
3. It has also been used in quantitative analysis. For example:
   The specific refraction of certain silicate glasses vary nearly linearly with the more percentage of LiO_2 over a range of 50–90% thus by measuring refractive index and density of the silicon content in such glasses can be easily calculated.

PRECAUTIONS

1. **Cleaning:** Clean the surfaces of prism with dry cotton, then clean them with distilled water, then with cotton dipped in acetone and lastly wipe off the surface with dry cotton.
2. **Temperature Constancy:** To maintain temperature, there must be inlet and outlet for rubber tubing so that water of constant temperature can run through it.
3. **Packing:** While packing the metal encasing, it should be kept in mind that no gap remains after packing.

By finding refractive index we can find adulteration of water in glycerin, and structure conformation is also possible.

PROCEDURE

1. Clean the surfaces of the prism with dry cotton and then clean with distilled water.
2. Again clean with acetone and finally wipe the surface with dry cotton.
3. Place a drop of pure benzene on the surface.
4. Now clamp the prism A and B in order to make a film between them.
5. View through the telescope in such a way that the field of view should be equally divided into light and dark portion.
6. It should be noted that the bright portion should coincide with the cross-wire of the telescope.
7. Note the reading and least-count on the scale.
8. Calculate the R.I. of the benzene.

OBSERVATIONS

Molecular weight of liquid (Benzene) = 78.11

1. Density of liquid (Benzene) = 0.881 gm/ml^3.
2. R.I. of benzene = 1.51 + (9 divisions × 0.001) = 1.519

CALCULATION

1. Molar Refractivity of Benzene (Practical)

$$R = \frac{n^2 - 1}{n^2 + 2} \times \frac{M}{d}$$

Where

$$M = 78.11$$
$$d = 0.881$$
$$n = 1.519$$

$$= \frac{(1.519)^2 - 1}{(1.519)^2 + 2} \times \frac{78.11}{0.881}$$

$$= \frac{2.307361 - 1}{2.307361 + 2} \times \frac{78.11}{0.881}$$

$$= \frac{1.30736}{4.307361} \times \frac{78.11}{0.881}$$

$$= 26.91$$

2. Molar Refractivity of Benzene (Theoretical)

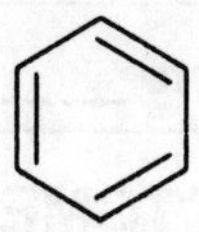

Molar refraction due to 6 C atoms	=	6 × 2.42	=	14.52
Molar refraction due to 6 H atoms	=	6 × 1.10	=	6.60
Molar refraction due to 3 double bonds	=	3 × 1.73	=	5.19
Molar refraction due to one six membered ring	=	1 × 0.15	=	0.15
		Total	=	26.46

DISCUSSION

Theoretical molar refraction (26.46) and practical molar refraction (26.91) values are fairly close, so the structure would be benzene only.

RESULT

The molar refraction of benzene was found to be 26.91.

EXPERIMENT 7.2B

Date ____________

MOLAR REFRACTION OF BENZENE BY ABBE'S REFRACTOMETER (Manual)

AIM

To find out the molar refraction of benzene by abbe's refractometer and also confirm the structure of benzene.

PROCEDURE

1. Clean the surfaces of the prism with dry cotton and then clean with distilled water.
2. Again clean with acetone and finally wipe the surface with dry cotton.
3. Place a drop of pure benzene on the surface.
4. Now clamp the prism A and B in order to make a film between them.
5. View through the telescope in such a way that the field of view should be equally divided into light and dark portion.
6. It should be noted that the bright portion should coincide with the cross-wire of the telescope.
7. Note the reading and least-count on the scale.
8. Calculate the R.I. of the benzene.

OBSERVATIONS

Molecular weight of liquid (Benzene) = 78.11

1. Density of liquid (Benzene) = 0.881 gm/ml^3
2. R.I. of Benzene = ________ + ________ divisions × 0.001

   = ________

CALCULATION

1. Molar Refractivity of Benzene (Practical)

$$R = \frac{n^2 - 1}{n^2 + 2} \times \frac{M}{d}$$

Where

M = 78.11

d = 0.881

n = ________

= ________ × ________

= ________ × ________

= ________ × ________

= ________

2. Molar Refractivity of Benzene (Theoretical)

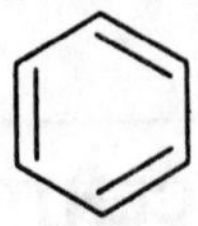

Molar refraction due to 6 C atoms	=	6 × 2.42	=	14.52
Molar refraction due to 6 H atoms	=	6 × 1.10	=	6.60
Molar refraction due to 3 double bonds	=	3 × 1.73	=	5.19
Molar refraction due to one six membered ring	=	1 × 0.15	=	0.15
			Total =	26.46

DISCUSSION

Theoretical molar refraction (26.46) and practical molar refraction (__________) values are fairly close, so structure would be benzene only.

RESULT

The molar refraction of benzene was found to be ________.

EXPERIMENT 7.3A

Date ____________

DETERMINATION OF CONCENTRATION OF GLYCERIN

AIM

To find out the concentration of unknown sample of glycerin by refractometry.

PRINCIPLE

When the beam of light is allowed to pass from rare (air) into denser medium such as liquid, the beam suffers refraction. According to Snell's law, the ratio of the sine of the angle of incidence and refraction is constant and is called as the refractive index of the liquid.

$$n = \frac{\sin i}{\sin r}$$

i = angle of incidence

r = angle of refraction

n is refractive index of the liquid.

The R.I. is a physical property of the liquids used to identify them.

CH_2OH
|
$CHOH$
|
CH_2OH

Glycerol

Mol. Formula: $C_3H_8O_3$ **Mol. Wt.:** 92.09

Glycerin is propane-1, 2, 3-triol.

Category: Lubricant; laxative; pharmaceutical aid (humectant).

Description: Clear, colourless or almost colourless, syrupy liquid; odourless; very hygroscopic.

Solubility: Miscible with water and with ethanol (95%); slightly soluble in acetone; practically insoluble in ether and in fixed oils and volatile oils.

ASSAY

Weigh accurately about 0.1 g, mix thoroughly with 45 ml of water, add 25.0 ml of a 2.14% w/v solution of sodium periodate and 1.0 ml of 1M sulphuric acid. Allow the mixture to stand protected from light for 15 minutes. Add 5 ml of a 50% w/v solution of ethylene glycol, allow to stand protected from light for 20 minutes and titrate with 0.1M sodium hydroxide using 0.5 ml of phenolphthalein solution as indicator. Repeat the procedure without the substance being examined. The differences between the titrations represent the amount of sodium hydroxide required by the test substance. Each ml of 0.1M sodium hydroxide is equivalent to 0.00921 g of $C_3H_8O_3$.

PROCEDURE

1. Take 0 ml, 2 ml, 4 ml, 6 ml, 8 ml and 10 ml quantity of glycerin in different test tubes.
2. Add distilled water in order to make the different concentration of glycerin 0%, 20%, 40%, 60%, 80% and 100% respectively by thorough mixing.
3. Clean the surfaces of the prism with dry cotton and then clean with distilled water.

4. Again clean with acetone and finally wipe the surface with dry cotton.
5. Place a drop of pure benzene on the surface.
6. Now clamp the prism A and B in order to make a film between them.
7. View through the telescope in such a way that the field of view should be equally dividing into light and dark portion.
8. It should be noted that the bright portion should coincide with the cross-wire of the telescope.
9. Note the reading and least-count on the scale.
10. Calculate the R.I. of the benzene.
11. Adopt the same procedure for all the solution as well as for unknown sample of which concentration is to be determined.
12. Plot a standard curve between the different known concentrations of glycerin *vs.* R.I.
13. Calculate the percentage of unknown sample of glycerin from the straight line.

OBSERVATION

S. No.	Different concentrations of glycerin in water	R.I.
1.	0%	1.379
2.	20%	1.403
3.	40%	1.436
4.	60%	1.467
5.	80%	1.478
6.	100%	1.570
7.	Unknown sample	1.445

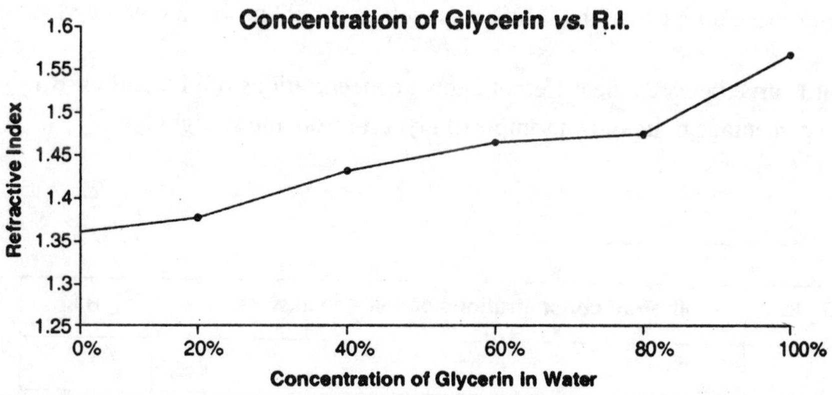

RESULT

The concentration of unknown sample of glycerin was found to be 42%.

EXPERIMENT 7.3B

Date ________

DETERMINATION OF CONCENTRATION OF GLYCERIN
(Manual)

AIM

To find out the concentration of unknown sample of glycerin by refractometry.

PROCEDURE

1. Take 0 ml, 2 ml, 4 ml, 6 ml, 8 ml and 10 ml quantity of glycerin in different test tubes.
2. Add distilled water in order to make the different concentration of glycerin 0%, 20%, 40%, 60%, 80% and 100% respectively by thorough mixing.
3. Clean the surfaces of the prism with dry cotton and then clean with distilled water.
4. Again clean with acetone and finally wipe the surface with dry cotton.
5. Place a drop of pure benzene on the surface.
6. Now clamp the prism *A* and *B* in order to make a film between them.
7. View through the telescope in such a way that the field of view should be equally dividing into light and dark portion.
8. It should be noted that the bright portion should coincide with the cross-wire of the telescope.
9. Note the reading and least-count on the scale.
10. Calculate the R.I. of the benzene.
11. Adopt the same procedure for all the solution as well as for unknown sample of which concentration is to be determined.
12. Plot a standard curve between the different known concentrations of glycerin *vs.* R.I.
13. Calculate the percentage of unknown sample of glycerin from the straight line.

OBSERVATION

S. No.	Different concentrations of glycerin in water	R.I.
1.	0%	
2.	20%	
3.	40%	
4.	60%	
5.	80%	
6.	100%	
7.	Unknown sample	

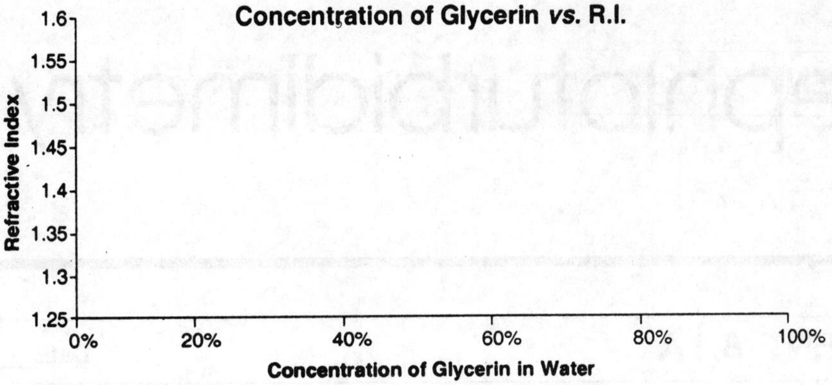

RESULT

The concentration of unknown sample of glycerin was found to be __________ %.

Nephloturbidimetry 8

EXPERIMENT 8.1 A

Date ____________

LIMIT TEST FOR CHLORIDE

AIM

To perform the limit test for chloride in the given solution by using nephloturbidimetry.

PRINCIPLE

Nephlometry and Turbidimetry are the instrumental techniques of analysis based upon the scattered and transmitted light by non-transparent particles suspended in a solution. When a light is allowed to pass through the solution, a part of radiation is absorbed, reflected and refracted, while the remaining is transmitted. The basis of turbidimetric analysis is the measurement of this transmitted light as a function of the concentration of the suspended particles.

The limit test for chloride can be performed with the help of Nephloturbidimetry as chloride can be determined as AgCl by Turbidimetry. The NTU of sample solution should be within the NTU of standard to pass the test for chloride.

PROCEDURE

1. **Preparation of standard opalescence**
   (*a*) Take 10 ml of chloride standard solution (25 ppm chloride) into a Nessler cylinder.
   (*b*) Add 10 ml of dilute nitric acid and make up the volume to 50 ml with distilled water (turbidity free).
   (*c*) Add 1 ml of 0.1N silver nitrate solution and stir immediately to produce the turbidity.
   (*d*) Allow it to stand for 5 minutes protected from light.
2. **Preparation of sample opalescence**
   (*a*) Pipette out 10 ml of sample solution into another Nessler cylinder.
   (*b*) Add 10 ml of dilute nitric acid and make up the volume to 50 ml with distilled water (turbidity free).
   (*c*) Add 1 ml of 0.1N silver nitrate and stir immediately.
   (*d*) Allow the resulting solution to stand for 5 minutes protected from light.
3. **Measurement of Nephloturbidimetric Unit (NTU)**
   (*a*) Switch on the instrument.
   (*b*) Allow it to stabilize for 10 minutes.
   (*c*) Place distilled water and adjust the reading to 0%.
   (*d*) Discard the water and take standard opalescence and adjust the reading to 100%.
   (*e*) Run sample opalescence and compare the percentage NTU with the standard opalescence.

OBSERVATION

S. No.	Preparation	NTU Range	Meter Reading	Total (NTU × meter reading)
1.	Standard solution	100	50	5,000
2.	Sample solution	100	26	2,600

RESULT

As the NTU meter reading of sample solution is lesser than standard NTU range, the given sample of chloride passes the limit test for chloride.

EXPERIMENT 8.1 B

Date ______

LIMIT TEST FOR CHLORIDE
(Manual)

AIM

To perform the limit test for chloride in the given solution by using nephloturbidimetry.

PROCEDURE

1. **Preparation of standard opalescence**
   (*a*) Take 10 ml of chloride standard solution (25 ppm chloride) into a Nessler cylinder.
   (*b*) Add 10 ml of dilute nitric acid and make up the volume to 50 ml with distilled water (turbidity free).
   (*c*) Add 1 ml of 0.1N silver nitrate solution and stir immediately to produce the turbidity.
   (*d*) Allow it to stand for 5 minutes protected from light.
2. **Preparation of sample opalescence**
   (*a*) Pipette out 10 ml of sample solution into Nessler cylinder.
   (*b*) Add 10 ml of dilute nitric acid and make up the volume to 50 ml with distilled water (turbidity free).
   (*c*) Add 1 ml of 0.1N silver nitrate and stir immediately.
   (*d*) Allow the resulting solution to stand for 5 minutes protected from light.
3. **Measurement of Nephloturbidimetric Unit (NTU)**
   (*a*) Switch on the instrument.
   (*b*) Allow it to stabilize for 10 minutes.
   (*c*) Place distilled water and adjust the reading to 0%.
   (*d*) Discard the water and take standard opalescence and adjust the reading to 100%.
   (*e*) Run sample opalescence and compare the percentage NTU with the standard opalescence.

OBSERVATION

S. No.	Preparation	NTU Range	Meter Reading	Total (NTU × meter reading)
1.	Standard solution			
2.	Sample solution			

RESULT

As the NTU meter reading of sample solution is greater/lesser than standard NTU range, therefore the given sample of chloride passes/does not pass the limit test for chloride.

EXPERIMENT 8.2 A

Date ____________

LIMIT TEST FOR SULPHATE

AIM

To perform the limit test for sulphate in the given solution by using nephloturbidimetry.

PRINCIPLE

Nephlometry and Turbidimetry are the instrumental techniques of analysis based upon the scattered and transmitted light by non-transparent particles suspended in a solution. When a light is allowed to pass through the solution, a part of radiation is absorbed, reflected and refracted; while the remaining is transmitted. The basis of turbidimetric analysis is the measurement of this transmitted light as a function of the concentration of the suspended particles. Sulphate determination in coke, coal, oils, rubber, plastics and other organic substance can be carried out with Nephloturbidimetry. In order to determine sulphur, firstly all the sulphur is converted into sulphate followed by shaking with sodium chloride and excess of solid barium chloride to get barium sulphate suspension.

PROCEDURE

A. Preparation of Standard Turbidity

1. Pipette out 1.5 ml of ethanolic standard sulphate solution into Nessler cylinder.
2. To this add 1 ml of 25% w/v barium chloride solution.
3. Mix and allow to stand for 1 minute.
4. To this add 15 ml of (10 ppm) standard sulphate solution and 0.15 ml of 5 M acetic acid.
5. Make up the volume to 50 ml with distilled water.
6. Stir immediately with glass rod and allow to stand for 5 minutes.

B. Preparation of Sample Turbidity

1. Pipette out 1.5 ml of ethanolic standard sulphate solution into Nessler cylinder.
2. Add 1 ml of 25% w/v barium chloride solution.
3. Mix and allow to stand for 1 minute.
4. To this solution, add 15 ml of sample solution.
5. Add 0.15 ml of 5 M acetic acid.
6. Make up the volume to 50 ml with distilled water.
7. Stir immediately and allow to stand for 10 minutes.

C. Measurement of Nephloturbidimetric Unit (NTU)

1. Switch on the instrument.
2. Allow it to stabilize for 10 minutes.
3. Place distilled water and adjust the reading to 0%.

4. Discard the water and take standard opalescence and adjust the reading to 100%.
5. Run sample opalescence and compare the percentage NTU with the standard opalescence.

OBSERVATION

S. No.	Preparation	NTU range	Meter reading	Total NTU × Meter reading
1.	Standard	1000	50	50,000
2.	Sample	1000	35	35,000

RESULT

As the NTU range × meter reading of the sample was found less than that of standard solution, therefore the given sample passes the limit test for sulphate.

EXPERIMENT 8.2B

Date ______

LIMIT TEST FOR SULPHATE
(Manual)

AIM

To perform the limit test for sulphate in the given solution by using nephloturbidimetry.

PROCEDURE

A. Preparation of Standard Turbidity

1. Pipette out 1.5 ml of ethanolic standard sulphate solution into Nessler cylinder.
2. To this add 1 ml of 25% w/v barium chloride solution.
3. Mix and allow to stand for 1 minute.
4. To this add 15 ml of (10 ppm) standard sulphate solution and 0.15 ml of 5 M acetic acid.
5. Make up the volume to 50 ml with distilled water.
6. Stir immediately with glass rod and allow to stand for 5 minutes.

B. Preparation of Sample Turbidity

1. Pipette out 1.5 ml of ethanolic standard sulphate solution into Nessler cylinder.
2. Add 1 ml of 25% w/v barium chloride solution.
3. Mix and allow to stand for 1 minute.
4. To this solution, add 15 ml of sample solution.
5. Add 0.15 ml of 5 M acetic acid.
6. Make up the volume to 50 ml with distilled water.
7. Stir immediately and allow to stand for 10 minutes.

C. Measurement of Nephloturbidimetric Unit (NTU)

1. Switch on the instrument.
2. Allow it to stabilize for 10 minutes.
3. Place distilled water and adjust the reading to 0%.
4. Discard the water and take standard opalescence and adjust the reading to 100%.
5. Run sample opalescence and compare the percentage NTU with the standard opalescence.

OBSERVATION

S. No.	Preparation	NTU range	Meter reading	Total NTU × Meter reading
1.	Standard			
2.	Sample			

RESULT

As the NTU range × meter reading of the sample was found greater/lesser than that of standard solution, therefore the given sample passes/does not pass the limit test for sulphate.

Chromatography (TLC, Paper, HPLC, HPTLC) 9

EXPERIMENT 9.1 A **Date** ______

THIN LAYER CHROMATOGRAPHY

AIM

To identify the given sample of amino acid with the help of thin layer chromatography and also calculate R_f value of individual amino acids.

THEORY

Chromatography is the separation and purification techniques employed for organic as well as for inorganic compounds. Two or more compounds or ions are separated by the distribution between two phases, one, which is moving, and the other, which is stationary. These two phases can be solid–liquid, liquid–liquid or gas–liquid.

Types of Chromatography

Chromatography is classified as follows:

1. **Gas Chromatography**
   (*a*) Gas–liquid chromatography
   (*b*) Gas–solid chromatography
2. **Liquid Chromatography**
   (*a*) Liquid–liquid chromatography
   (*b*) Liquid–solid chromatography
   (*c*) Ion exchange chromatography
   (*d*) Exclusion chromatography

Physical surface forces are mainly involved in the retentive ability of the stationary phase in most of the chromatographic procedures. When the stationary phase is liquid and mobile phase is either liquid or gas, the process is called partition chromatography. In contrast, when the stationary phase is solid and mobile phase is either liquid or gas, it is categorized under adsorption type of chromatography.

Two other liquid chromatographic methods differ somewhat in their mode of action. For example, in ion exchange chromatography (IEC), ionic components of the sample are separated by selective exchange with ions of the stationary phase. Exclusion chromatography (EC) is referred to or gel permeation chromatography by polymer chemists and as gel filtration by biochemists.

THIN LAYER CHROMATOGRAPHY (TLC)

Thin – layer chromatography or TLC is a solid–liquid form of chromatography where the stationary phase is normally a polar absorbent, usually finely ground alumina or silica particles. This absorbent is coated on a glass slide or plastic sheet creating a thin layer of the particular stationary phase. By manipulating the mobile phase, organic compounds can be separated. The mobile phase can be a single solvent or combination of solvents. TLC is a quick, inexpensive micro scale technique that can be used to:

- determine the number of components in a mixture,
- verify a substance's identity,
- monitor the progress of a reaction,
- determine appropriate conditions for column chromatography and
- analyze the fractions obtained from column chromatography.

Stationary Phase

As stationary phase, a special finely ground matrix (silica gel, alumina or similar material) is coated on a glass plate, a metal or a plastic film as a thin layer (~0.25 mm in thickness). In addition, a binder like gypsum as in Silica gel G is mixed into the stationary phase to make it stick better to the slide. In many cases, a fluorescent powder is mixed into the stationary phase to simplify the visualization later on (e.g. bright green when we expose it to 254 nm UV light). Uniform thin layer of adsorbent is placed on the support by various techniques. These are mainly:

(*a*) Spreading

(*b*) Dipping

(*c*) Spraying

After placement of layer of adsorbent, the plate is dried in air for 5–10 minutes and then in oven for half an hour at 110° C temperature.

Preparing the plate

In order to obtain an imaginary start line with pencil, make two notches on each side of the TLC plate.

Capillary spotters

Place a melting point capillary in the dark blue part of the Bunsen burner flame. Hold it there until it softens and starts to sag. Quickly remove the capillary from the flame and pull on both ends to about 2-3 times its original length. Allow the capillary to cool down, and then break it in the middle. Make sure that you break off the closed end on one of them.

Spotting of the TLC plate

One advantage TLC has over other separation methods is that it is truly a micro scale technique. Only a few micrograms of material in solution is necessary to observe the solute on a TLC plate. Dissolve a few milligrams of material in a solvent (preferably volatile) creating a dilute solution. Once the sample is prepared, a spotting capillary must be used to add the sample to the plate. The solution can be drawn up in the tube by capillary action and spotted on the plate at the place marked by pencil. This is known as the origin.

Pencil is always used to mark a TLC plate since the graphite carbon is inert. To spot the plate, simply touch the end of the capillary tube to the coated side of the plate. The solvent should evaporate quickly leaving the mixture behind on the plate. You may have to spot the plate a couple of times to ensure the material present, but do not spot too much sample. If too much solute is added to the plate, a poor separation will result. Smearing, smudging and spots that overlap will result making identification of separated components difficult.

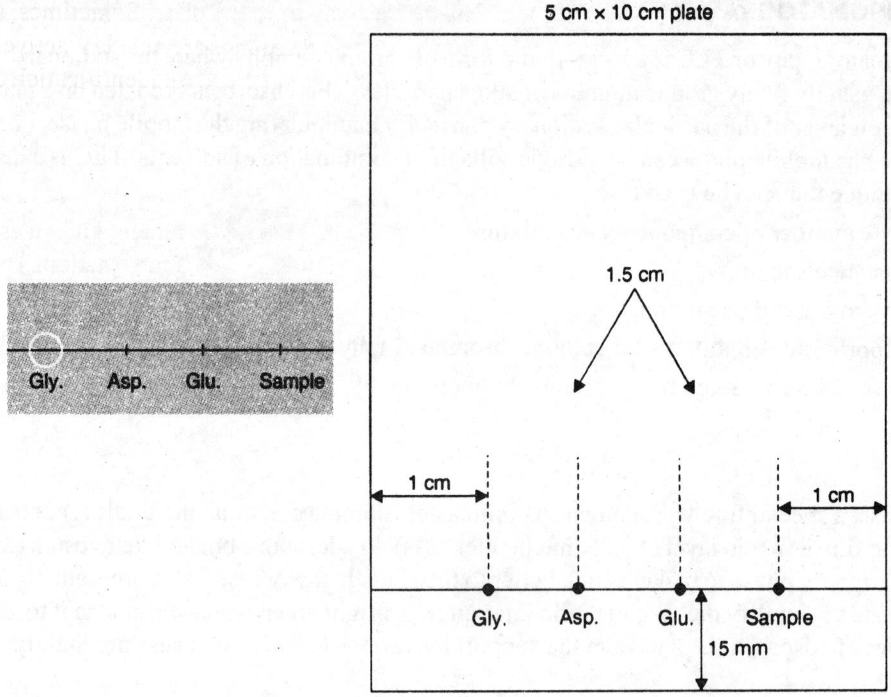

Development

Once the dilute solution of the mixture has been spotted on the plate, the next step is the development of the plate. The bottle (chamber) is filled with a small amount of the mobile phase and covers it. In addition, a piece of filter paper is put in the chamber to help create an atmosphere saturated with solvent. Also make sure, the origin spots are not below the solvent level in the chamber. If the spots are submerged in the solvent, they are washed off the plate and lost.

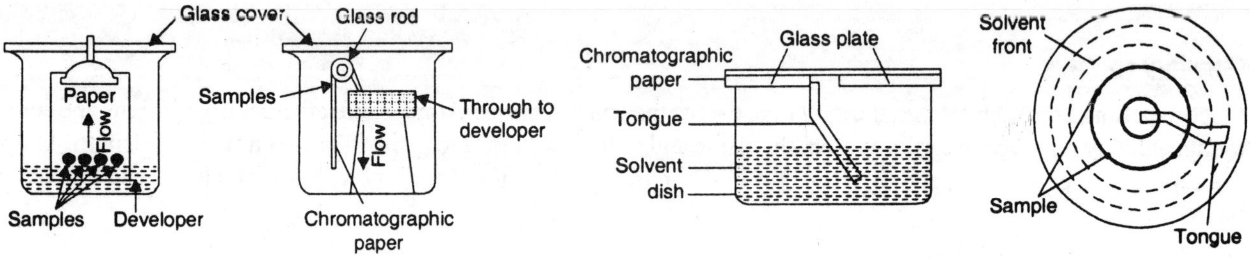

Visualization

If organic compounds are coloured such as dyes, inks or indicators, then visualization of the separated spots is easy. However, since most organic compounds are colourless, this method does not work.

In most cases observing the separated spots by UV light works well. TLC plates normally contain a fluorescent indicator which makes the TLC plate glow green under UV light of wavelength 254 nm. Compounds that absorb UV light, will quench the green fluorescence yielding dark purple or bluish spots on the plate. Simply put the plate under a UV lamp, and the compounds become visible to the naked eye. Lightly circle the spots to have a permanent record of their location for later calculations.

Another useful visualizing technique is an iodine (I_2) chamber. Iodine sublimes and will absorb organic molecules in the vapour phase. The organic spots on the plate will turn brown and can be easily identified. Also circle these observed spots, since the iodine adsorbed spots eventually fade away from the plate. Sometimes, a combination of both a UV lamp and iodine is needed to observe all the spots. Some compounds are not "UV active", that is, they do not absorb light at the wavelength of 254 nm. Using both methods will ensure correct identification of all the spots on the TLC plate.

R_f Value

In addition to qualitative results, TLC can also provide a chromatographic measurement known as an R_f value. The R_f value is the "retardation factor" or the "ratio-to-front" value expressed as a decimal fraction. The R_f value can be calculated as:

$$R_f \text{ value} = \frac{\text{Distance from the origin to centre of spot}}{\text{Distance from the origin to solvent front}}$$

This number can be calculated for each spot observed on a TLC plate. Essentially it describes the distance traveled by the individual components. If two spots travel the same distance or have the same R_f value then it might be concluded that the two components are the same molecule. For R_f value comparisons to be valid; however, TLC plates must be run under the same exact conditions. These conditions include the stationary phase, mobile phase, and temperature. Just as many organic molecules have the same melting point and colour, many can have the same R_f value, so identical R_f values doesn't necessarily mean identical compounds. Additional information must be obtained before this conclusion can be made. It is important to restate that R_f value is only significant when the same chromatographic conditions are used.

Solution

Prepare a 0.5 or 1% solution of standard amino acid like glycine, aspartic acid, glutamic acid etc., in water or ethanol. Similarly prepare a solution of unknown amino acid which is to be identified.

Developer

Prepare a mixture of glacial acetic acid, water and 1-butanol in a proportion of 20, 20 and 60 by volume.

Spraying agent

Prepare a 0.2% Ninhydrin solution in 95 volume of 1-butanol and 5 volume of acetic acid.

PROCEDURE

1. Clean the glass plate (support for adsorbent).
2. Make a suspension or slurry of silica gel *G* in distilled water and spread on given size plate that is rested on an absolutely labeled surface. Spread the slurry or suspension on the surface of plate by the backward and forward movement.
3. Dry the plate at room temperature for 5–10 minutes and then in oven at 110° C for half an hour.
4. Meanwhile prepare a mobile phase (developer) and pour into jar. Place a filter paper around the wall of jar. Cover the jar properly and allow to saturate the jar with the vapours of mobile phase for better development.
5. Draw an imaginary start-line with pencil, make two notches on each side of the TLC plate.
6. Draw a solution with the help of capillary and simply touch the end of the capillary tube to the coated side of the plate for spotting. Allow the solvent to evaporate quickly leaving amino acid behind on the plate. Spot the plate a couple of times to ensure the material present, but do not spot too much sample. Like this, spot the probable amino acid and unknown amino acid on the same imaginary line on the plate with 1 cm apart.
7. Insert the plate in the developing chamber containing mobile phase but make sure, the origin spots are not below the solvent level in the chamber. If the spots are submerged in the solvent, they will be washed off the plate and lost.

8. Take out the plate gently when the mobile phase is about to touch the upper side of the plate. Mark the solvent front with pencil and dry the plate in well ventilated area or in oven.
9. Spray the plate with spraying agent, dry the plate in oven and mark the spot.
10. Calculate the R_f value and compare the R_f value of unknown amino acid with standard amino acid.

OBSERVATION

S. No.	Amino acid	Distance traveled by amino acid	Distance traveled by solvent front	R_f value
1.	Glycine	3.7 cm	10 cm	0.37
2.	Aspartic acid	2.4 cm	10 cm	0.24
3.	Glutamic acid	1.8 cm	10 cm	0.18
4.	**Unknown**	**2.5 cm**	**10 cm**	**0.25**

RESULT

On the basis of same R_f value, the unknown amino acid was found to be aspartic acid.

EXPERIMENT 9.1 B

Date ____________

THIN LAYER CHROMATOGRAPHY
(Manual)

AIM

To identify the given sample of amino acid with the help of thin layer chromatography and also calculate R_f value of individual amino acids.

PROCEDURE

1. Clean the glass plate (support for adsorbent).
2. Make a suspension or slurry of silica gel *G* in distilled water and spread on given size plate that is rested on an absolutely labeled surface. Spread the slurry or suspension on the surface of plate by the backward and forward movement.
3. Dry the plate at room temperature for 5–10 minutes and then in oven at 110° C for half an hour.
4. Meanwhile prepare a mobile phase (developer) and pour into jar. Place a filter paper around the wall of jar. Cover the jar properly and allow to saturate the jar with the vapours of mobile phase for better development.
5. Draw an imaginary start-line with pencil, make two notches on each side of the TLC plate.
6. Draw a solution with the help of capillary and simply touch the end of the capillary tube to the coated side of the plate for spotting. Allow the solvent to evaporate quickly leaving amino acid behind on the plate. Spot the plate a couple of times to ensure the material present, but do not spot too much sample. Like this, spot the probable amino acid and unknown amino acid on the same imaginary line on the plate with 1 cm apart.
7. Insert the plate in the developing chamber containing mobile phase but make sure the origin spots are not below the solvent level in the chamber. If the spots are submerged in the solvent, they will be washed off the plate and lost.
8. Take out the plate gently when the mobile phase is about to touch the upper side of the plate. Mark the solvent front with pencil and dry the plate in well ventilated area or in oven.
9. Spray the plate with spraying agent, dry the plate in oven and mark the spot.
10. Calculate the R_f value and compare the R_f value of unknown amino acid with standard amino acid.

OBSERVATION

S. No.	Amino acid	Distance traveled by amino acid	Distance traveled by solvent front	R_f value
1.	Glycine			
2.	Aspartic acid			
3.	Glutamic acid			
4.	Unknown			

RESULT

On the basis of same R_f value, the unknown amino acid was found to be ____________

EXPERIMENT 9.2 A

Date ____________

THIN LAYER CHROMATOGRAPHY

AIM

To identify the given drug amongst the paracetamol, aspirin and caffeine citrate with the help of thin layer chromatography and calculate its R_f value.

CHROMATOGRAPHIC CONDITIONS

Standard Solution: Prepare a 0.5 or 1% solution of Paracetamol, Aspirin and Caffeine citrate in methanol.

Sample Solution: Prepare the sample solution by dissolving in methanol, followed by sonication and centrifugation.

Mobile Phase: Ethyl acetate: Glacial acetic acid (95:5)

Detecting Agent: U.V. or Iodine chamber.

OBSERVATION

S. No.	Amino acid	Distance traveled by amino acid	Distance traveled by solvent front	R_f value
1.	Paracetamol	4.8 cm	10 cm	0.48
2.	Aspirin	6.7 cm	10 cm	0.67
3.	Caffeine citrate	2.4 cm	10 cm	0.24
4.	**Unknown**	**4.6 cm**	**10 cm**	**0.46**

RESULT

On the basis of same R_f value, the unknown sample was found to be Paracetamol.

EXPERIMENT 9.2 B

Date ____________

THIN LAYER CHROMATOGRAPHY
(Manual)

AIM

To identify the given drug amongst the paracetamol, aspirin and caffeine citrate with the help of thin layer chromatography and calculate its R_f value.

Chromatographic Conditions

Standard Solution: Prepare a 0.5 or 1% solution of Paracetamol, Aspirin and Caffeine citrate in methanol.

Sample Solution: Prepare the sample solution by dissolving in methanol, followed by sonication and centrifugation.

Mobile Phase: Ethyl acetate : Glacial acetic acid (95:5)

Detecting Agent: U.V. or Iodine chamber.

OBSERVATION

S. No.	Amino acid	Distance traveled by amino acid	Distance traveled by solvent front	R_f value
1.	Paracetamol			
2.	Aspirin			
3.	Caffeine citrate			
4.	Unknown			

RESULT

On the basis of same R_f value, the unknown sample was found to be ____________________.

EXPERIMENT 9.3A

Date ______

THIN LAYER CHROMATOGRAPHY

AIM

To identify the given sulpha drug among the sulphadiazine, sulphamethoxazole and trimethoprim with the help of thin layer chromatography and calculate its R_f value.

Solution

Prepare a 0.5 or 1% solution of Sulphadiazine, Sulphamethoxazole, Trimethoprim and unknown sulpha drug in methanol.

Developer

Prepare a mixture of chloroform and methanol in 90 and 9.5 proportions by volume.

Visualizing agent: U.V. or Iodine chamber.

PROCEDURE

It is similar to Experiment 9.1 but in this, keep the developed plate after drying in UV chamber. Mark the brown coloured spot and calculate the R_f value and compare the R_f value of unknown drug with Sulphadiazine, Sulphamethoxazole and Trimethoprim.

OBSERVATION

S. No.	Amino acid	Distance traveled by amino acid	Distance traveled by solvent front	R_f value
1.	Sulphadiazine	0.3 cm	10 cm	0.03
2.	Sulphamethoxazole	4.9 cm	10 cm	0.49
3.	Trimethoprim	2.4 cm	10 cm	0.24
4.	Unknown	4.8 cm	10 cm	0.48

RESULT

On the basis of same R_f value, the unknown sample is found to be Sulphamethoxazole.

EXPERIMENT 9.3B

Date ____________

THIN LAYER CHROMATOGRAPHY
(Manual)

AIM

To identify the given sulpha drug among the sulphadiazine, sulphamethoxazole and trimethoprim with the help of thin layer chromatography and calculate its R_f value.

Solution

Prepare a 0.5 or 1% solution of Sulphadiazine, Sulphamethoxazole, Trimethoprim and unknown sulpha drug in methanol.

Developer

Prepare a mixture of chloroform and methanol in 90 and 9.5 proportions by volume.

Visualizing agent: U.V. or Iodine chamber.

PROCEDURE

It is similar to Experiment 9.1 but in this, keep the developed plate after drying in UV chamber. Mark the brown coloured spot and calculate the R_f value and compare the R_f value of unknown drug with Sulphadiazine, Sulphamethoxazole and Trimethoprim.

OBSERVATION

S. No.	Amino acid	Distance traveled by amino acid	Distance traveled by solvent front	R_f value
1.	Sulphadiazine			
2.	Sulphamethoxazole			
3.	Trimethoprim			
4.	Unknown			

RESULT

On the basis of same R_f value, the unknown sample is found to be ____________.

EXPERIMENT 9.4A

Date ____________

PAPER CHROMATOGRAPHY

AIM

To perform the separation of amino acids by paper chromatography.

PRINCIPLE

Paper chromatography is a technique in which the principle of separation is partition. Whatmann filter paper acts as stationary phase (because the filter paper contains moisture in its cellulose layers) and organic solvents or mixture employed as mobile phase.

PROCEDURE

1. **Preparation of solutions of amino acids**
   (*a*) Make 0.1% solution of amino acids, glycine, phenyl (alanine and Proline) in mobile phase.
   (*b*) Now take any two solutions 1 ml each and mix them thoroughly and use as sample mixture.
   (*c*) Label all the solutions.
2. **Preparation of mobile phase (developing solvent)**
   (*a*) Mix 40 ml *n*-butanol, 10 ml glacial acetic acid and 50 ml water in a separating funnel.
   (*b*) Shake the mixture thoroughly and allow to separate.
   (*c*) Use aqueous layer as developing solvent or mobile phase.
3. **Preparation of visualizing (Ninhydrin reagent)**
   Take 2 gm of ninhydrin in 100 ml *n*-butanol and fill it in a spray bottle.
4. Take Whatmann filter paper of (25 × 5 cm) and draw a thin straight line about 5–6 cm above from the bottom edge of the paper.
5. Now mark 4 points at equal distance and label these as G, PA, P and S(sample).
6. With the help of capillary tubes apply the solution of amino acids and sample mixture as well on the specified marks of the filter paper. It is to be noted that the drop must be as compact as possible and allow these spots to dryness.
7. Pour the mobile phase in the chromatographic chamber and allow saturating for 30 minutes with the help of filter paper.
8. Hang the filter paper containing spots in the chamber in such a manner that it should just touch the surface of the solvent.
9. Cover the chamber and allow the solvent to rise to about 3/4th height of the paper.
10. Remove this paper and draw a line to make the solvent front.
11. Dry this chromatogram in air for at least 9–10 minutes.
12. Spray the ninhydrin solution on it and again dry in hot air oven at 50–55° C for 15 minutes, purple colour spots will visualize.
13. The pure amino acids will have a single spot and in case of sample mixture to separate spots will be obtained as the mixture contains two amino acids.
14. Measure the distances of the developed spots and solvent front.
15. Calculate the R_f values of each separated amino acid and compare with the R_f values of pure amino acid.

OBSERVATION

S. No.	Amino acid	Distance traveled by amino acid	Distance traveled by solvent front	R_f value
1.	Glycine	3.6 cm	10 cm	0.36
2.	Phenyl alanine	2.6 cm	10 cm	0.26
3.	Proline	1.2 cm	10 cm	0.12
4.	Unknown	1.3 and 3.5 cm	10 cm	0.13 and 0.35

RESULT

On the basis of same R_f value, the unknown sample is found to be the mixture of Glycine and Proline.

EXPERIMENT 9.4B

Date ____________

PAPER CHROMATOGRAPHY
(Manual)

AIM

To perform the separation of amino acids by paper chromatography.

PROCEDURE

1. **Preparation of solutions of amino acids**
   (*a*) Make 0.1% solution of amino acids (Glycine, Phenyl alanine and Proline) in mobile phase.
   (*b*) Now take any two solutions 1 ml each and mix them thoroughly and use as sample mixture.
   (*c*) Label all the solutions.
2. **Preparation of mobile phase (developing solvent)**
   (*a*) Mix 40 ml *n*-butanol, 10 ml glacial acetic acid and 50 ml water in a separating funnel.
   (*b*) Shake the mixture thoroughly and allow to separate.
   (*c*) Use aqueous layer as developing solvent or mobile phase.
3. **Preparation of visualizing (Ninhydrin reagent)**
   Take 2 gm of Ninhydrin (Triketo hydrindene hydrate) in 100 ml *n*-butanol and fill it in a spray bottle.
4. Take Whatmann filter paper of (25 × 5 cm) and draw a thin straight line about 5–6 cm above from the bottom edge of the paper.
5. Now mark 4 points at equal distance and label these as G, PA, P and S (sample).
6. With the help of capillary tubes, apply the solution of amino acids and sample mixture as well on the specified marks of the filter paper. It is to be noted that the drop must be as compact as possible and allow these spots to dryness.
7. Pour the mobile phase in the chromatographic chamber and allow saturating for 30 minutes with the help of filter paper.
8. Hang the filter paper containing spots in the chamber in such a manner that it should just touch the surface of the solvent.
9. Cover the chamber and allow the solvent to rise to about 3/4th height of the paper.
10. Remove this paper and draw a line to make the solvent front.
11. Dry this chromatogram in air for at least 9–10 minutes.
12. Spray the Ninhydrin solution on it and again dry in hot air oven at 50–55° C for 15 minutes, purple colour spots will visualize.
13. The pure amino acids will have a single spot and in case of sample mixture to separate spots will be obtained as the mixture contains two amino acids.
14. Measure the distances of the developed spots and solvent front.
15. Calculate the R_f values of each separated amino acid and compare with the R_f values of pure amino acid.

OBSERVATION

S. No.	Amino acid	Distance traveled by amino acid	Distance traveled by solvent front	R_f value
1.	Glycine			
2.	Phenyl alanine			
3.	Proline			
4.	Unknown			

RESULT

On the basis of same R_f value, the unknown sample is found to be the mixture of ____________________.

EXPERIMENT 9.5A

Date ______

PAPER CHROMATOGRAPHY

AIM

To identify the given sample of sugar with the help of ascending paper chromatography and calculate its R_f value.

PRINCIPLE

Paper chromatography is a technique in which the analysis of unknown substances is carried out mainly by the flow of solvents on specially designed filter paper. There are two types of paper chromatography.

(*i*) Paper adsorption chromatograph in which paper impregnated with silica or alumina act as adsorbent (stationary phases) and solvent as mobile phases.

(*ii*) Paper partition chromatograph in which moisture/water present in the pores of cellulose fibers present in filter paper act as stationary phases and another mobile phase is used as solvent.

In general, paper chromatograph refers to paper partition chromatograph only since most separations are based on partition type only.

Principles of Separation

Paper chromatography is, in the general principle, quite similar to thin-layer chromatography. As in TLC, R_f values are often used to characterize compounds separated by a given solvent and absorbent combination, and are, in fact, even more reproducible and widely used. The main differences between the two techniques are:

1. The use of paper (i.e. cellulose fibers) as absorbent;
2. Lack of backing as support; and
3. The use of more polar solvents for separation of more polar constituents.

The principle of separation is mainly partition rather than adsorption. A cellulose layer in filter paper contains moisture that act as stationary phase. Organic solvents or buffers are used as mobile phases. Instead of water as stationary phase, other organic solvents can be used by suitable modification.

Chromatographic paper is available most commonly in 20 cm × 20 cm sheets. The underlying principle behind the use of paper as a absorbent is that water molecules that associate with cellulose fibers interact with molecules in the mobile phase via hydrogen bonding. As a result, more polar molecules are resolved by PC, and more polar solvents are employed. In addition to solvent, the use of an electric field has been employed in so-called paper electrophoresis.

In addition, descent paper chromatography in which solvent is provided to the top of the chromatogram has been widely employed. Other variations include circular or horizontal paper chromatography for which apparatuses are available.

Stationary Phase

Cut a piece of chromatographic paper to fit into the development chamber of particular size. Mark a line on the bottom edge of the paper with the help of pencil. On this line, spotting of the sample has to be done. Sample spots must be made by pencil on the chromatography paper.

For very crude separations, separations can be done using high-grade filter paper as the stationary phase. Paper of chromatographic grade consists of α-cellulose 98.99%, β-cellulose 0.3%, pentosans 0.4–0.8%, ether soluble matter 0.015–0.02%, ash 0.01–0.07%. Whatmann filter papers of different grade like No. 1, No. 2, No. 3, No. 4, No. 17, No. 20 etc. are used. These papers differ in sizes, shape, porosities and thickness. Choice of filter paper depends upon thickness flow rate, purity and technique etc.

Development

Choose a developing chamber that can be sealed well. The chamber should be large enough to hold the paper that is to be developed. Add the mobile phase to the chamber so that it is about 2 cm deep. Seal the chamber tightly and let the chamber stand until the atmosphere becomes saturated. A saturated atmosphere allows for more effective development of the chromatograms.

Mobile Phase

Pure solvents, buffer solutions or mixtures of solvents are used. Some of the examples of hydrophilic mobile phase:

Isopropanol : liquid ammonia : water (9 : 1 : 2)

n-butanol : glacial acetic acid : water (4 : 1 : 5)

Methanol : water (3 : 1 or 4 : 1)

t-butanol : water : formic acid (40 : 20 :5)

Loading of the Sample on the Paper

Each sample should be dissolved in an appropriate solvent to make about a-one percent solution. Less than one millilitre of solution is required for the experiment. Touch the tip of a clean drawn-out capillary tube to the sample and let about 3 mm of the sample rise into the tube. If too much solution is drawn into the capillary, touch the tip to a piece of clean filter paper. To spot the sample, touch the capillary to the line (as marked with pencil) on the chromatogram. Make sure, the spot does not exceed 1 cm in diameter. Allow the solvent to evaporate. More than one sample can be loaded onto a single piece of chromatography paper. However, all spots on the chromatogram should be 2–2.5 cm away from the edges of the paper and from each other.

If a larger quantity of sample is needed for the experiment than is provided by one application, the solution may be respotted. When the original spot has dried, draw solution into the capillary as before. Apply this solution over the top of the first spot, but do not allow the diameter of the circle to grow larger than that of the original spot. Repeat it if necessary, allowing each spot to dry before the next application.

Development of the Chromatogram

After preparing the chamber and spotting the samples, the paper is ready to be developed. Be careful to handle the paper only by its edges to prevent contamination. Initially, the chromatogram should be suspended in the chamber without touching the solvent. To suspend the chromatogram, thread a piece of string through a paper clip at the top of it. Then tape the string to the outside of the chamber to hold the chromatogram in place. After the chromatogram has hung in the chamber for 10 minutes, immerse the paper's bottom edge into the developing solvent.

Ascending Development

Like conventional type, the solvent flows against gravity. The spots are kept at the bottom portion of paper and kept in a chamber with mobile phase solvent at the bottom. In a chromatographic chamber, the solvent rises up the paper by capillary action and allows a separation of the components as it ascends. Very simple equipments are required. However, the solvent will rise only 20–25 cm and separations of the analytes are limited.

Descending Development

This is carried out in a special chamber where the solvent holder is at the top. The spot is kept at the top and the solvent flows down the paper. The advantage is that the flow of solvent is assisted by gravity and hence the development is faster.

In a chromatographic chamber, a paper strip is hanged vertically with the spotted end-up. The solvent rises up the wick and descends across the spot and down the paper. This technique permits a separation over a longer distance and allows an increase in resolution.

Ascending–Descending Development

This is a combination of ascending and descending type. Only using a combination of techniques increases the length of separation. First ascending takes place followed by descending development.

Circular/Radial Development (Horizontal)

Here the spot is kept at the centre of a circular paper. The solvent flows through a wick at the centre and spread in all directions uniformly. Hence, the individual look like concentric circles. By making perforations radically, number of quadrants can be created allowing more number of samples to be spotted.

Two-dimensional Development

The paper is developed in the second direction allowing more compounds or complex mixtures, either the same solvent system or different system can be used for development. A solution of interested is subjected to two separation processes in two-dimensional technique. A sample solution is spotted in one corner of a square or rectangular sheet of paper. One solvent is applied to separate the analytes in one direction. After the paper is dried and turned 90° and developed in a second solvent, high degree of separation of the analytes can be achieved by this technique.

Removing the Chromatogram

After the solvent front is within half an inch of the top of the paper, remove the chromatogram. First, open the lid of the development chamber. Then gently lift the string and the chromatogram out of the chamber. Be sure to handle the chromatogram only by the sides. Carefully mark the solvent front with a pencil and allow the chromatogram to dry in a well-ventilated area.

Visualization of the Spots

After the chromatogram has dried, one can identify the spots. Detect the coloured spots visually. If the spots can be seen, outline them with a pencil. Sometimes the colour will fade overtime, so the pencil outline is important. If the spots are not visible, the most common visualization technique is to hold the paper under an ultraviolet lamp. (Caution: Do not look directly into the lamp!) Many organic compounds can be seen using this technique. Outline the spots with a pencil, while the chromatogram is under the UV lamp.

Non-specific methods: In this, the number of spots can be detected, but not the exact nature of type of compound.

Iodine chamber method: In this, brown or amber spots are observed when the paper is kept in a closed jar containing few iodine crystals at the bottom.

Specific methods: Specific spray reagents, detecting agents or visualizing agents are used to find out the nature of compounds or for identification purposes.

Examples:

Ferric chloride—for phenolic compounds and tannins.

Ninhydrin in acetone—for amino acids.

Dragendroff reagents—for alkaloids.

3, 5-dinitro benzoic acid—for cardiac glycosides.

2, 4-dinitrophenyl hydrazine—for aldehydes and ketones.

The detecting techniques can also be categorized as;

Destructive technique: e.g. Specific spray reagents, etc. where the samples are destroyed before detection. e.g. Ninhydrin reagents.

Non-destructive technique: Like UV chamber method, iodine chamber method, densitometry method, etc. where the samples is not destroyed even after detection.

Interpreting the Chromatogram

The R_f value for each spot should be calculated. It is characteristic for any given compound on the same stationary phase, using the same mobile phase for development of the chromatogram. Hence, known R_f values can be compared to those of unknown substances to aid in their identifications.

$$R_f \text{ values} = \frac{\text{Distance from the origin to centre of spot}}{\text{Distance from the origin to solvent front}}$$

Note: R_f values often depend on the temperature, solvent, and type of paper used in the Experiment No. 9.4; the most effective way to identify a compound is to spot known substances next to unknown substances on the same chromatogram.

In addition, the purity of a sample may be estimated from the chromatogram. An impure sample will often develop as two or more spots.

Solution

Prepare a 0.5 or 1% solution of standard sugar like glucose, fructose, sucrose etc., in water or ethanol.

Similarly prepare a solution of unknown sugar which is to be identified.

Developer

Prepare a mixture of *n*-butanol, pyridine and water in a proportion of 6:4:3 by volume.

Spraying agent

Dissolve phthalic acid (1.66 gm) and aniline (0.9 ml) in *n*-butanol (48 ml) and mix with ether (48 ml) and water (4 ml).

PROCEDURE

1. Cut a strip of Whatmann No. 1 chromatographic paper (30–40 cm × 5 cm).
2. Draw a line about 2″ from the top of the paper with pencil and draw four small circles on the line with pencil on the lower side of sheet and mark these as *G* for glucose, *F* for fructose, *S* for sucrose and *U* for unknown sugar.
3. Touch the tip of a clean drawn out capillary tube to the sample solution of glucose and let about 3 mm of the sample rise into the tube. To spot the sample, touch the capillary to the marked circle on the chromatogram. Make sure, the spot does not exceed 1 cm in diameter. Allow the solvent to evaporate. Similarly spot the other solution at respective circle. However, all spots on the chromatogram should be 2–2.5 cm away from the edges of the paper and from each other.
4. Fill the chamber with developer (mobile phase), close the chamber with cover and allow to remain undisturbed for 15 minutes for proper saturation. After preparing the chamber and spotting the samples, the paper is ready to be developed. Be careful to handle the paper only by its edges to prevent contamination. Initially, suspend the chromatogram in the chamber containing mobile phase without dipping the spotted marks.
5. Allow the paper to develop till the mobile phase just reaches the other end of the paper.

6. Take out the paper gently, carefully mark the solvent front with a pencil and allow the chromatogram to dry in a well-ventilated area.
7. Spray the chromatogram with spraying reagent and dry in oven to visualize the brownish spot.
8. Calculate the R_f value of each sugar molecule.

OBSERVATION

S.No.	Sugar	Distance traveled by amino acid	Distance traveled by solvent front	R_f value
1.	Glucose	0.3 cm	10 cm	0.03
2.	Fructose	4.9 cm	10 cm	0.49
3.	Sucrose	2.4 cm	10 cm	0.24
4.	Unknown	4.8 cm	10 cm	0.48

RESULT

On the basis of R_f value, the unknown sugar is found to be fructose.

EXPERIMENT 9.5 B

Date ______________

PAPER CHROMATOGRAPHY
(Manual)

AIM

To identify the given sample of sugar with the help of ascending paper chromatography and calculate its R_f value.

PROCEDURE

1. Cut a strip of Whatmann No. 1 chromatographic paper (30–40 cm × 5 cm).
2. Draw a line about 2″ from the top of the paper with pencil and draw four small circles on the line with pencil on the lower side of sheet and mark these as G for glucose, F for fructose, S for sucrose and U for unknown sugar.
3. Touch the tip of a clean drawn-out capillary tube to the sample solution of glucose and let about 3 mm of the sample rise into the tube. To spot the sample, touch the capillary to the marked circle on the chromatogram. Make sure, the spot does not exceed 1 cm in diameter. Allow the solvent to evaporate. Similarly spot the other solution at respective circle. However, all spots on the chromatogram should be 2–2.5 cm away from the edges of the paper and from each other.
4. Fill the chamber with developer (mobile phase), close the chamber with cover and allow to remain undisturbed for 15 minutes for proper saturation. After preparing the chamber and spotting the samples, the paper is ready to be developed. Be careful to handle the paper only by its edges to prevent contamination. Initially, suspend the chromatogram in the chamber containing mobile phase without dipping the spotted marks.
5. Allow the paper to develop, till the mobile phase just reaches the other end of the paper.
6. Take out the paper gently, carefully mark the solvent front with a pencil and allow the chromatogram to dry in a well-ventilated area.
7. Spray the chromatogram with spraying reagent and dry in oven to visualize the brownish spot.
8. Calculate the R_f value of each sugar molecule.

OBSERVATION

S. No.	Sugar	Distance traveled by amino acid	Distance traveled by solvent front	R_f value
1.	Glucose			
2.	Fructose			
3.	Sucrose			
4.	Unknown			

RESULT

On the basis of R_f value, the unknown sugar is found to be ______________

EXPERIMENT 9.6

Date ____________

HIGH PERFORMANCE LIQUID CHROMATOGRAPHY

AIM

To demonstrate high performance liquid chromatography.

PRINCIPLE

High performance liquid chromatography is based upon the principle of absorption. It is modified technique of column chromatography and also called as high pressure liquid chromatography.

The high performance is because of the superior separation of the components due to the wide surface area provided for absorption. The particle size of the silica gel is about 0.5 μ. The use of pump makes the technique faster and various types of detectors can be used to analyze the components.

The different parts of high performance liquid chromatography are:

1. Solvent reservoirs—To store for mobile phase.
2. Pumps—To maintain the flow rate of mobile phase.
3. Sample injector—To inject the sample into the mobile phase.
4. Guard column—To saturate the mobile phase with silica and to guard the analytical column from impurities/ particles.
5. Analytical column—To carry out the separation of the components from the complex mixture by absorption technique.
6. Detector—To analyze the components, separate from the columns.
7. Readont—To plot the chromatograms.

The high performance liquid chromatography is of two modes:

1. Normal phase
2. Reverse phase

1. **Normal phase mode:** In this mode, the stationary phase is polar in nature while the mobile phase is non-polar. The non-polar components travel faster and eluted first, while the polar components take more time to elute.
2. **Reverse phase mode:** In this mode, the stationary phase is non-polar and the mobile phase is polar in nature. The polar components elute faster and non-polar components take more time to elute. Since most of the pharmaceutical drugs are polar in nature, this technique is largely used for analytical purpose.

PROCEDURE

1. Prepare mobile phase.
2. Prepare sample solution containing the mixture of the components to be separated.
3. Switch on the instrument.
4. Place the mobile phase into the solvent reservoir.
5. Turn on the pumps and set the flow rate as specified in the selected method.
6. Maintain the pressure within the limits as per the column used.
7. Turn on the detector and wait for 5 min. for stabilization.
8. Set the λ_{max}/detection wavelength.
9. Run the mobile phase for at least 10 minutes.

10. Correct the baseline for 10 minutes. Connect the detector for mobile phase.
11. Inject the sample solution into the sample injector and allow the sample to run for specified run time.
12. Analyze the chromatogram for different components.

The identification of the eluted components can be carried out by comparing the retention time of the component with that of standard. The quantity of the component present can be carried out by various methods:

I. Direct comparison method

By comparing the peak areas of sample and standard solutions, the quantity of the sample can be determined.

$$\text{Peak area} = \text{Peak height} \times \text{Peak width}$$

$$\frac{A_1}{A_2} = \alpha \frac{C_1}{C_2}$$

A_1 and A_2 are peak areas of sample and standard.

C_1 and C_2 are concentrations of sample and standard

α = Response factor.

II. Calibration curve method

For a series of standard solutions with different concentrations, plot the curve taking concentration on x-axis and peak area on y-axis. Extrapolate the peak area of sample to find out the concentration.

EXPERIMENT 9.7 A

Date ____________

HIGH PERFORMANCE THIN LIQUID CHROMATOGRAPHY

AIM

To analyze the given tablets of paracetamol/ibuprofen–paracetamol combination by HPTLC method.

PRINCIPLE

INTRODUCTION

HPTLC (High Performance Thin Layer Chromatography) is a sophisticated and automated form of TLC. The main difference of HPTLC and TLC is particle and pore size of absorbents. The differences are:

	HPTLC	TLC
Layer of absorbent	100 µm	250 µm
Efficiency	High due to smaller particle size generated in HPTLC	Less
Separations	3–5 cm	10–15 cm
Analysis time	Shorter migration distance and the analysis time is greatly reduced for HPTLC and is faster than TLC	
Solid support	Wide choice of stationary phases like silica gel for normal phase and C_8, C_{18} for reversed phase modes (HPTLC)	Silica gel, Alumina and Kiesulgur
Development chamber	New type that require less amount of mobile phase	More amount
Sample spotting	Auto sampler	Manual spotting
Scanning	Use of UV/Visible/Fluorescence scanner scans the entire chromatogram qualitatively and quantitatively and the scanner is an advanced type of densitometer	Not possible

Features of HPTLC

1. Simultaneous processing of sample and standard—better analytical precision and accuracy—less need for Internal standard.
2. Several analysts work simultaneously.
3. Lower analysis time and less cost per analysis.
4. Low maintenance cost.
5. Simple sample preparation—handle samples of divergent nature.
6. No prior treatment for solvents like filtration and degassing.
7. Low mobile phase consumption per sample.

8. No interference from previous analysis—fresh stationary and mobile phases for each analysis—no contamination.
9. Visual detection possible — open system.
10. Non UV absorbing compounds detected by post-chromatographic derivatization.

Steps Involved in HPTLC

- Selection of chromatographic layer
- Sample and standard preparation
- Layer pre-washing
- Layer pre-conditioning
- Application of sample and standard
- Chromatographic development
- Detection of spots
- Scanning
- Documentation of chromatoplate

Selection of Chromatographic Layer

- Precoated plates — different support materials — different absorbents available
- 80% of analysis — silica gel GF
- Basic substances, alkaloids and steroids — aluminium oxide
- Amino acids, dipeptides, sugars and alkaloids — cellulose
- Non-polar substances, fatty acids, carotenoids, cholesterol — RP_2, RP_8 and RP_{18}
- Preservatives, barbiturates, analgesic and phenothiazines — hybrid plates-$RPWF_{254s}$

Sample and Standard Preparation

- Normal Phase Mode — Non-polar solvent should be used for dissolving the sample and standard.
- Reverse Phase Mode — Polar solvent should be used for dissolving the sample and standard.

Layer Pre-washing

- To avoid interference from impurities and water vapours
- Low signal to noise ratio — Straight base line — Improvement of LOD
- Solvents used are Methanol, Chloroform : Methanol (1:1), Ethyl acetate : Methanol (1:1), Chloroform : Methanol : Ammonia (90:10:1), Methylene chloride : Methanol (1:1), 1% Ammonia or 1% Acetic acid
- Dry the plates and store in dust free atmosphere

Activation of Pre-coated Plates

- Freshly open box of plates do not require activation.
- Plates exposed to high humidity or kept on hand for long time to be activated.
- By placing in an oven at 110–120° C for 30 minutes prior to spotting.
- Aluminium sheets should be kept in between two glass plates and placing in oven at 110–120° C for 15 minutes.

Application of Sample and Standard

- Usual concentration range is 0.1–1 µg/µl
- Above this causes poor separation

- Linomat IV (automatic applicator) — nitrogen gas sprays sample and standard from syringe on TLC plates as bands
- Band wise application — better separation — high response to densitometer

Selection of Mobile Phase

- Trial and error
- One's own experience and Literature
- Normal phase — Stationary phase is polar
- Mobile phase is non-polar
- Non-polar compounds eluted first because of lower affinity with stationary phase
- Polar compounds retained because of higher affinity with the stationary phase
- Reversed phase — Stationary phase is non-polar
- Mobile phase is polar
- Polar compounds eluted first because of lower affinity with stationary phase
- Non-polar compounds retained because of higher affinity with the stationary phase
- 3–4 component mobile phase should be avoided
- Multi component mobile phase once used not recommended for further use and solvent composition is expressed by volumes (v/v) and sum of volumes is usually 100
- Twin trough chambers are used — only 10–15 ml of mobile phase is required
- Components of mobile phase should be mixed — introduced into the twin–trough chamber

Pre-conditioning (Chamber saturation)

- Un-saturated chamber causes high R_f values
- Saturated chamber by lining with filter paper for 30 minutes prior to development — uniform distribution of solvent vapours — less solvent for the sample to travel — lower R_f values

Chromatographic Development and Drying

- After development, remove the plate and mobile phase is removed from the plate — to avoid contamination of lab atmosphere
- Dry in vacuum desiccator — avoid hair drier — essential oil components may evaporate

Detection and Visualization

- Detection under UV light is first choice — non-destructive.
- Spots of fluorescent compounds can be seen at 254 nm (short wavelength) or at 366 nm (long wavelength).
- Spots of non fluorescent compounds can be seen — fluorescent stationary phase is used — silica gel GF.
- Non UV absorbing compounds like ethambutol, dicyclomine etc—dipping the plates in 0.1% iodine solution.
- When individual component does not respond to UV derivatization required for detection.

Quantification

- Sample and standard should be chromatographed on same plate — after development chromatogram is scanned.
- Camag TLC scanner III scan the chromatogram in reflectance or in transmittance mode by absorbance or by fluorescent mode — scanning speed is selectable up to 100 mm/s — spectra recording is fast — 36 tracks with up to 100 peak windows can be evaluated.

- Calibration of single and multiple levels with linear or non-linear regressions are possible
- When target values are to be verified such as stability testing and dissolution profile, single level calibration is suitable
- Statistics such as RSD or CI report automatically
- Concentration of analyte in the sample is calculated by considering the sample initially taken and dilution factors

Documentation

E-Merck introduced plates with imprinted identification code — supplier name. Item number, batch number and individual plate number — avoid manipulation of data at any stage — coding automatically gets recorded during photo documentation.

Validation of Analytical Method

All validation parameters such as precision, accuracy, LOD, LOQ, ruggedness, robustness can be performed

PROCEDURE

About instrument: High performance liquid chromatograph (Merk, Hitachi, model D-7000) equipped with dual reciprocal pump (L-7100) monitor LG, Rheodyne injector folding a 20 µl loop licrosol RP-8 column fitted with a licrosol RP-8 pre-column. The detector is equipped with 254 nm filter.

Chromatographic conditions: The mobile phase was filtered through 0.45 µm filter (Whatmann). The column was conditioned with a mobile phase till a stable base line was obtained. Mobile phase contains acetonitrile : water for HPLC (1:1) and pH was adjusted at 3.3 with acetic acid (HPLC grade). The flow rate of mobile phase was 1–2 ml/min. at which pressure remains constant nearly 50–51 bars.

Calibration curve for Ibuprofen and Paracetamol: Standard solutions representing 2–10 µg/20 µl was prepared separately in mobile phase and filtered through 0.45 µm filter before injection. Calibration curve of both drugs were prepared by plotting peak curve area *vs.* drug concentrations.

Sample preparation: Ten marketed tablets each containing 500 mg drug was weighed accurately and triturates to get fine powder. The powder equivalent to 2–10 µg/20 µl of Ibuprofen and Paracetamol extracted with 10 ml of mobile phase and filtered through 0.45 µm filter prior to injection.

OBSERVATIONS

Standard curve of Paracetamol

Concentration (µg/20 µl)	Retention Time	Peak Area × 1000
2	2.19	190.8036
4	2.18	490.6260
6	2.24	854.5264
8	2.20	1190.2640
10	2.23	1393.7372

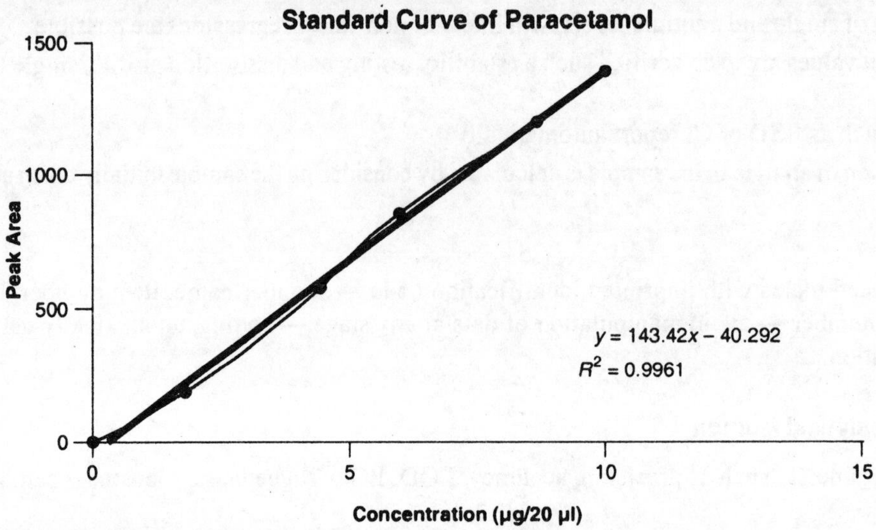

Standard Curve of Ibuprofen

Concentration (μg/20 μl)	Retention Time	Peak Area × 1000
2	6.8	174.80
4	6.9	382.62
6	6.8	648.52
8	6.7	890.26
10	6.8	1093.73

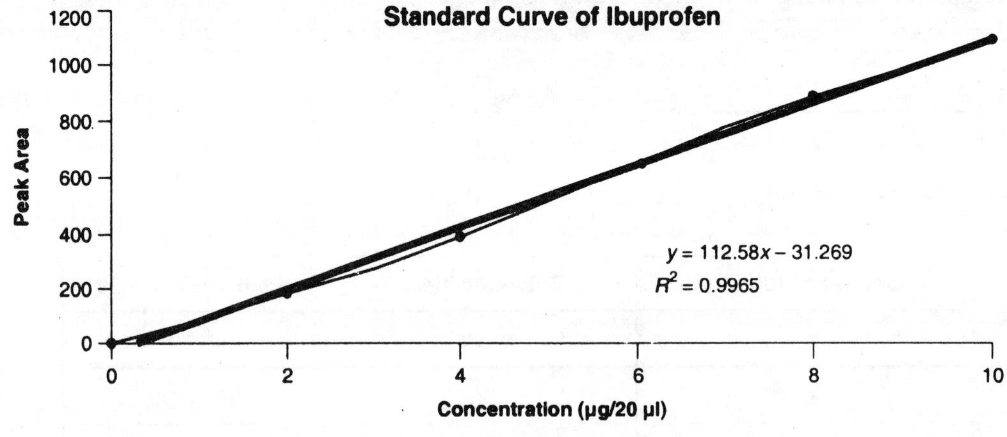

CALCULATION

$$R^2 = 0.99932$$
$$y = mx + c$$

$$y = 16289\,x - 6882$$

$$= \frac{-1237 + 6882}{16289}$$

$$= 7.81\ \mu g/20\ \mu l$$

Quantity of Paracetamol present in tablet

$$\frac{y - 6822}{16280} \times \text{Dilution factor} \times \frac{1}{1000}$$

$$\text{Labeled amount of Paracetamol} = \frac{9375.282 - 6882}{16280} \times \frac{10}{3} \times \frac{100}{2} \times 100 \times \frac{1}{1000}$$

$$= 95.85\%$$

$$\text{Labeled amount of Paracetamol} = 500\ \text{mg/Tablet}$$

$$\text{Given tablet contains} = \frac{95.85 \times 1000}{100} = 479.25\ \text{mg/Tablet}$$

Quantity of !buprofen present in tablet

$$\frac{y - 24.6}{124.95} \times \frac{10}{3} \times \text{Dilution factor} \times \frac{1}{1000}$$

$$\frac{1102 - 24.6}{124.95} \times \frac{10}{3} \times \frac{100}{3} \times 100 \times \frac{1}{1000} = 103.7\%$$

$$\text{Labeled amount of Ibuprofen} = 400\ \text{mg/Tablet}$$

$$\text{Given tablet contains} = \frac{103.7 \times 100}{100}$$

$$= 414.8\ \text{mg/Tablet}$$

RESULT

The Paracetamol/Ibuprofen combination tablet contains Paracetamol 479.25 mg/tablet (95.85%) and Ibuprofen 414.8 mg/tablet (103.7%).

EXPERIMENT 9.7 B

Date ____________

HIGH PERFORMANCE THIN LIQUID CHROMATOGRAPHY
(Manual)

AIM

To analyze the given tablets of paracetamol/ibuprofen–paracetamol combination by HPTLC method.

PROCEDURE

About Instrument: High performance liquid chromatograph (Merk, Hitachi, model D-7000) equipped with dual reciprocal pump (L-7100) monitor LG, Rheodyne injector folding a 20µl loop licrosol RP-8 column fitted with a licrosol RP-8 pre-column. The detector is equipped with 254 nm filter.

Chromatographic conditions: The mobile phase was filtered through 0.45 µm filter (Whatmann). The column was conditioned with a mobile phase till a stable base line was obtained. Mobile phase contains acetonitrile : water for HPTLC (1:1) and pH was adjusted at 3.3 with acetic acid (HPTLC grade). The flow rate of mobile phase was 1–2 ml/min. at which pressure remains constant nearly 50–51 bars.

Calibration curve for Ibuprofen and Paracetamol: Standard solutions representing 2–10 µg/20 µl was prepared separately in mobile phase and filtered through 0.45 µm filter before injection. Calibration curve of both drugs were prepared by plotting peak curve area *vs.* drug concentrations.

Sample preparation: Ten marketed tablets each containing 500 mg drug was weighed accurately and triturates to get fine powder. The powder equivalent to 2–10 µg/20 µl of Ibuprofen and Paracetamol extracted with 10 ml of mobile phase and filtered through 0.45 µm filter prior to injection.

OBSERVATIONS

Standard curve of Paracetamol

Concentration (µg/20 µl)	Retention Time	Peak Area × 1000
2		
4		
6		
8		
10		

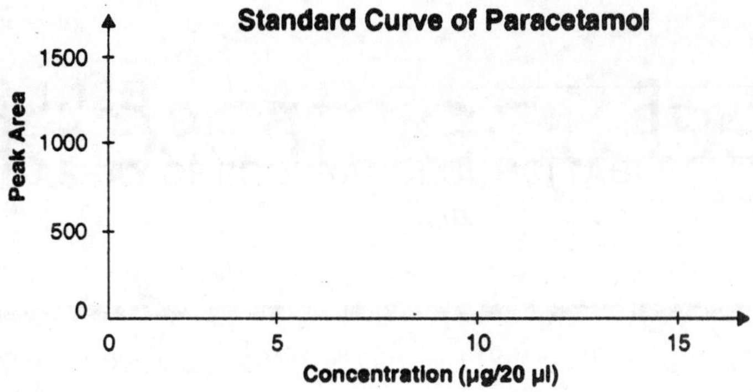

Standard Curve of Ibuprofen

Concentration (µg/20 µl)	Retention Time	Peak Area × 1000
2		
4		
6		
8		
10		

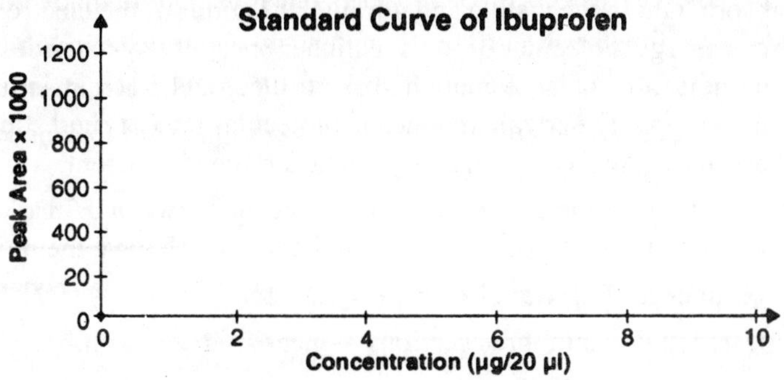

CALCULATION

R^2 = ___________

$y = mx + c$

y = __________ µg/20 µl

Quantity of Paracetamol present in tablet

Labeled amount of Paracetamol = 500 mg/Tablet

Given tablet contains = ______________________mg/Tablet

Quantity of Ibuprofen present in tablet

Labeled amount of Ibuprofen = 400 mg/Tablet

Given tablet contains = __________ mg/Tablet

RESULT

The Paracetamol/Ibuprofen combination tablet contains Paracetamol __________mg/Tablet (__________%) and Ibuprofen __________ mg/Tablet (__________%).

Infrared Spectroscopy 10

EXPERIMENT 10.1

Date ____________

INTERPRETATION OF INFRARED SPECTRA (A Practical Approach)

INTRODUCTION

The qualitative aspects of infrared spectroscopy are one of the most powerful attributes of this diverse and versatile analytical technique for the determination of functional groups in pure compounds and mixtures and for compounds comparison.

The organic compounds absorb light in the visible and ultraviolet regions of the electromagnetic spectrum when electrons are excited from lower energy molecular orbitals to higher ones. Photon energies associated with this part of the infrared (from 1–15 kcal/mole) are not large enough to excite electrons, but may induce vibrational excitation of covalently bonded atoms and groups. The covalent bonds in molecules are not rigid sticks or rods, such as found in molecular model kits, but are more like stiff springs that can be stretched and bent.

The term "infrared" covers the range of the electromagnetic spectrum between 0.78 and 1000 nm. In the context of infrared spectroscopy, wavelength is measured in "wave numbers", which have the units cm^{-1}.

Wave number = 1/Wavelength in centimeters

It is useful to divide the infrared region into three sections — near, mid and far infrared.

The most useful I.R. region lies between 4000–670 cm^{-1}.

Region	Wavelength (λ) range (μm)	Wave number range (cm^{-1})
Near	0.78–2.5	12800–4000
Middle	2.5–50	4000–200
Far	50–1000	200–10
Mostly used	2.5–15	4000–670
Finger print region		1300–400

Theory of Infrared Absorption

IR radiation does not have enough energy to induce electronic transitions as seen with UV. Absorption of IR is restricted to compounds with small energy differences in the possible vibrational and rotational states.

For a molecule to absorb IR, the vibrations or rotations within a molecule must cause a net change in the dipole moment of the molecule. The alternating electrical field of the radiation (remember that electromagnetic radiation consists of an oscillating electrical field and an oscillating magnetic field, perpendicular to each other) interacts with fluctuations in the dipole moment of the molecule. If the frequency of the radiation matches the vibrational frequency of the molecule, then radiation will be absorbed, causing a change in the amplitude of molecular vibration.

Molecular Rotations

Rotational levels are quantized, and absorption of IR by gases yields line spectra. However, in liquids or solids, these lines broaden into a continuum due to molecular collisions and other interactions.

Molecular Vibrations

The positions of atoms in a molecule are not fixed; they are subject to a number of different vibrations. Vibrations fall into the two main categories of stretching and bending.

Stretching: Change in inter-atomic distance along bond axis

Stretching vibrations

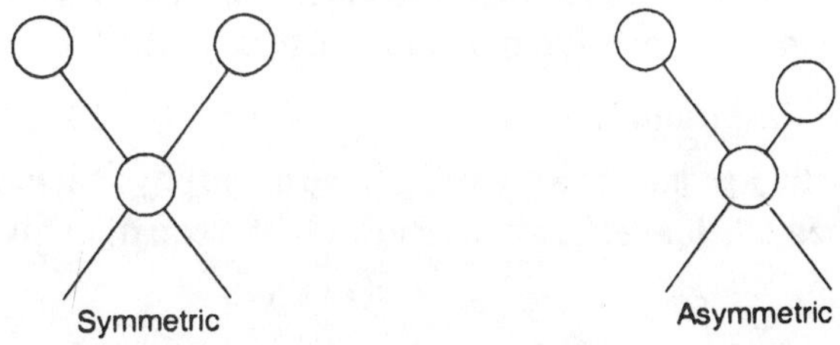

Bending: Change in angle between two bonds. There are four types of bending:

- Rocking
- Scissoring
- Wagging
- Twisting

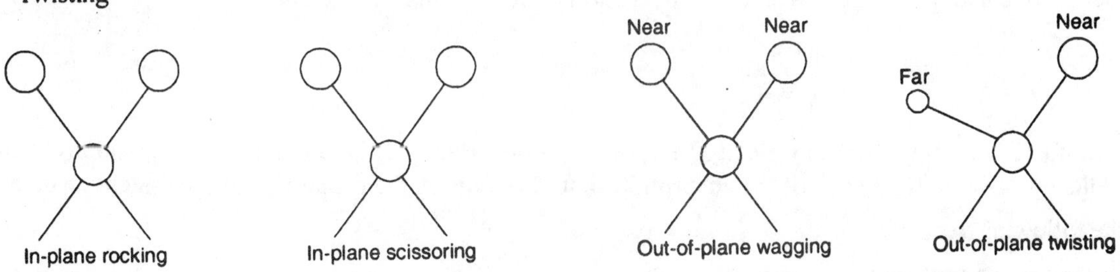

Vibrational Coupling

In addition to the vibrations mentioned above, interaction between vibrations can occur (coupling) if the vibrating bonds are joined to a single, central atom. Vibrational coupling is influenced by a number of factors;

- Strong coupling of stretching vibrations occurs when there is a common atom between the two vibrating bonds
- Coupling of bending vibrations occurs when there is a common bond between vibrating groups
- Coupling between a stretching vibration and a bending vibration occurs if the stretching bond is one side of an angle varied by bending vibration
- Coupling is greatest when the coupled groups have approximately equal energies
- No coupling is seen between groups separated by two or more bonds

Origin	Wavelength, λ	Frequency, ν (Wave numbers, cm^{-1})	Energy, Kcal/mole
Near infrared	0.8–2.5μ	12,500–400	35.7–11.4
Vibrational infrared	2.5–25μ	4000–400	11.4–1.14
Far infrared	0.025–0.5 mm	400–200	1.14–0.57

THE ORIGIN OF SPECTRUM

The infrared spectrum is formed as a consequence of the absorption of electromagnetic radiation at frequencies that correlate to the vibration of specific sets of chemical bonds from within a molecule. When seen the distribution of energy possessed by a molecule at any given moment, defined as the sum of the contributing energy are written as:

$$E_{total} = E_{electronic} + E_{vibrational} + E_{rotational} + E_{translational}$$

The translational energy relates to the displacement of molecules in space as a function of the normal thermal motions of matter. Rotational energy is observed as the tumbling motion of a molecule, which is the result of the absorption of energy within microwave region. The vibrational energy component is a higher energy term and corresponds to the absorption of energy by a molecule as the component atoms vibrate about the mean centre of their chemical bonds. The electronic component is linked to the energy transition of electrons as they are distributed throughout the molecule, either localized within specific bonds or delocalized over structures.

The position of infrared absorption band is specified in frequency units by its wave number measured in reciprocal centimeters (cm^{-1}) or by its wavelength, λ, measured in micrometers (μm).

$$V = 1/\lambda \text{ (with } \lambda \text{ in cm)} \quad \text{or} \quad V = 10{,}000/\lambda \text{ (with } \lambda \text{ in } \mu\text{m)}$$

To help understand IR, it is useful to compare a vibrating bond to the physical model of a vibrating spring system. The spring system can be described by Hooke's Law, as shown in the equation given below.

$$\nu = \frac{1}{2\pi}\sqrt{\frac{k}{\mu}}$$

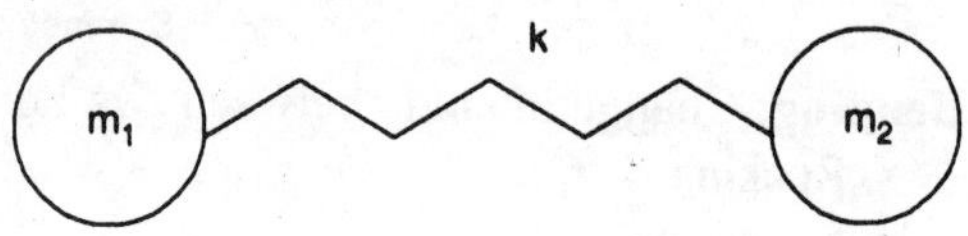

ν = frequency

μ = reduced mass

Consider a bond and the connected atoms to be a spring with two masses attached.

$$\mu = \frac{m_1 \cdot m_2}{m_1 + m_2}$$

Using the force constant *k* (which reflects the stiffness of the spring) and the two masses m_1 and m_2, then the equation indicates how the frequency of the absorption should change as the properties of the system change. Consider the following trends:

1. **For a stronger bond (larger *k* value)**

   As examples of this, in order of *increasing bond strength* compare:

   CC bonds: C—C (1000 cm^{-1}), C=C (1600 cm^{-1}) and C (2200 cm^{-1})

   CH bonds: C—C—H (2900 cm^{-1}), C=C—H (3100 cm^{-1}) and C—H (3300 cm^{-1})

   (*n.b.* make sure that you understand the bond strengths order)

2. **For heavier atoms attached**

   As examples of this, in order of *increasing reduced mass* compare:

   C—H (3000 cm^{-1})
   C—C (1000 cm^{-1})
   C—Cl (800 cm^{-1})
   C—Br (550 cm^{-1})
   C—I (about 500 cm^{-1})

The following diagram reflects some of the trends that can be accounted for using **Hooke's Law. It also gives** an approximate outline of where specific types of bond stretches may be found.

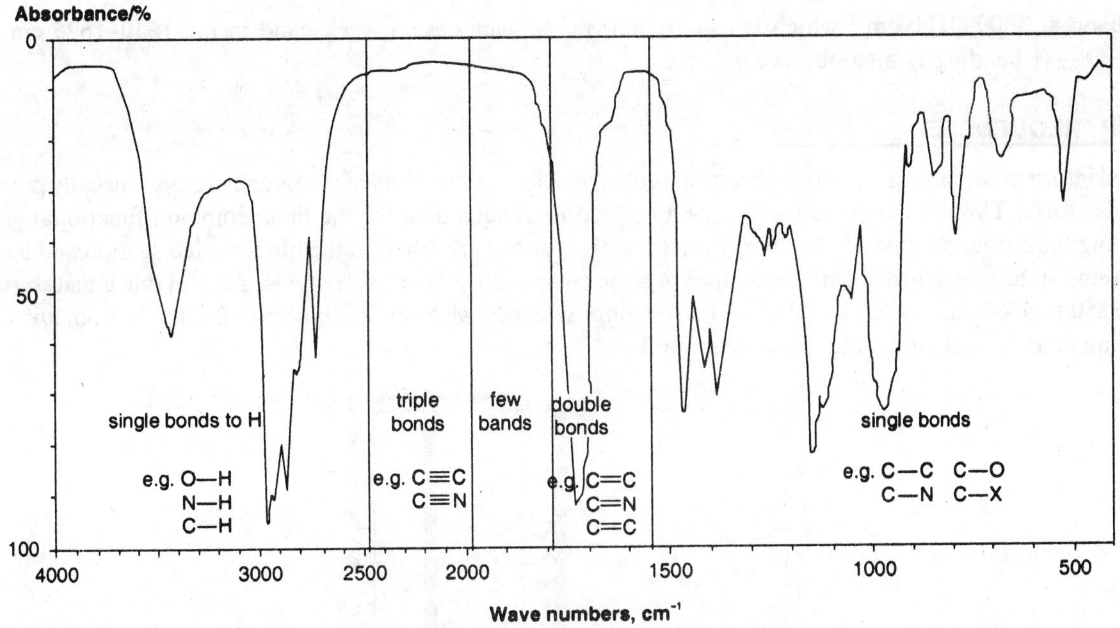

The general regions of the infrared spectrum in which various kinds of vibrational bands are observed are outlined in the following chart. Note that the blue coloured sections above the dashed line refer to stretching vibrations, and the green coloured band below the line encompasses bending vibrations. The complexity of infrared spectra in the 1450 to 600 cm^{-1} region makes it difficult to assign all the absorption bands, and because of the unique patterns found there, it is often called the **fingerprint** region. Absorption bands in the 4000 to 1450 cm^{-1} region are usually due to stretching vibrations of diatomic units, and this is sometimes called the **group frequency** region.

FUNDAMENTAL VIBRATIONS

A molecule composed of *n*-atoms has 3*n* degrees of freedom, six of which are translations and rotations of the molecule itself. This leaves $3n - 6$ degrees of vibrational freedom ($3n - 5$, if the molecule is linear). Vibrational modes are often given descriptive names, such as stretching, bending, scissoring, rocking and twisting. The four-atom molecule of formaldehyde, the gas phase spectrum of which is shown below, provides an example of these terms. If a ball and stick model of formaldehyde is not displayed to the right of the spectrum, press the **view ball and *n* stick model** button at the lower right. We expect six fundamental vibrations (12 minus 6), and these have been assigned to the spectrum absorptions.

SAMPLE HANDLING

Infrared spectra may be obtained from samples in all phases (liquid, solid and gaseous). Liquids are usually examined as a thin film sandwiched between two polished salt plates (note that glass absorbs infrared radiation, whereas NaCl is transparent). If solvents are used to dissolve solids, care must be taken to avoid obscuring important spectral regions by solvent absorption. Perchlorinated solvents such as carbon tetrachloride, chloroform and tetrachloroethene are commonly used. Alternatively, solids may either be incorporated in a thin KBr disk, prepared under high pressure, or mixed with a little non-volatile liquid and ground to a paste (or mull) that is smeared between salt plates.

SPECIAL CAUTIONS DURING SCANNING

Many spectra show a band at different region, such as band at 2350 cm^{-1} due to CO_2, when working room is not well-ventilated. Traces of moisture cause absorption around 3700 cm^{-1} which could be mistaken for a hydroxyl band. When IR perform for recrystallized sample, presence of water of crystallization gives rise to weak band at 3600–3100 cm^{-1} which is usually narrow. In such case a week band in the 1640–1625 cm^{-1} due to H—O—H bending is also observed.

GROUP FREQUENCIES

Detailed information about the infrared absorptions observed for various bonded atoms and groups is usually presented in tabular form. The following table provides a collection of such data for the most common functional groups. Following the colour scheme of the chart, stretching absorptions are listed in the blue-shaded section and bending absorptions in the green shaded part. Since most organic compounds have C—H bonds, a useful rule is that absorption in the 2850 to 3000 cm^{-1} is due to sp^3 C—H stretching; whereas, absorption above 3000 cm^{-1} is from sp^2 C—H stretching or sp C—H stretching if it is near 3300 cm^{-1}.

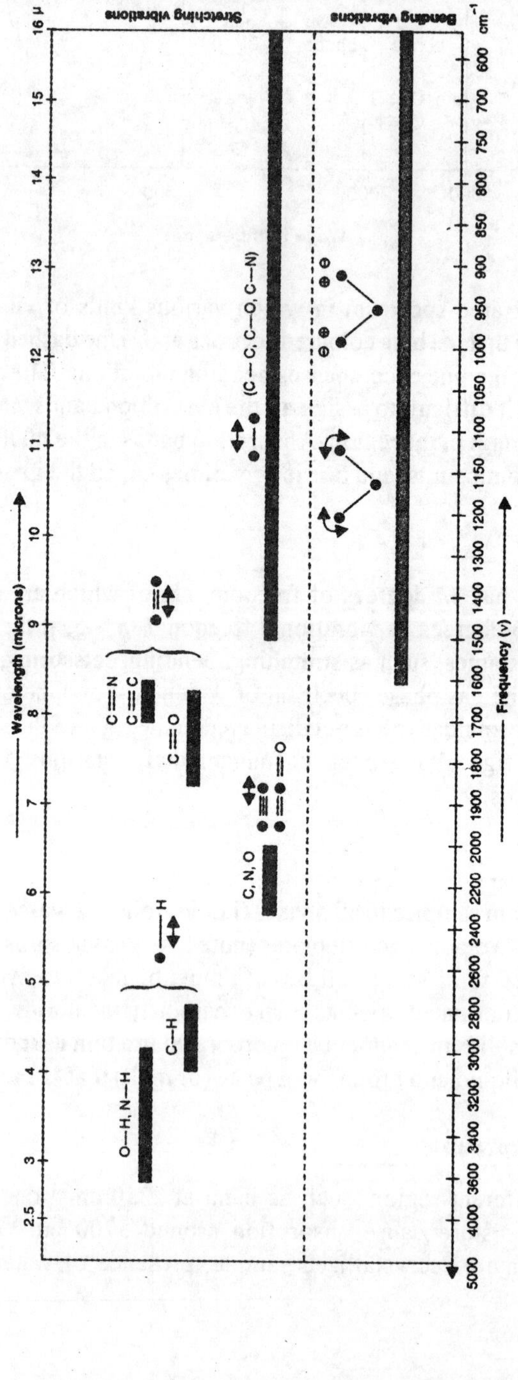

Typical Infrared Absorption Frequencies

	Stretching Vibrations			Bending Vibrations		
Functional Class	Range (cm^{-1})	Intensity	Assignment	Range (cm^{-1})	Intensity	Assignment
Alkanes	2970–2950/2880–2860 2935–2915/2815–2845 2850–2815	str	—CH_3(C—H asym/sym.) =CH_2 (C—H asym/sym.,) & CH special methyl like methoxy, methyl ether	1470–1430/1380–1350 1300–700 750–720	med wk	CH_2 and CH_3 asym/sym bend skeletal C—C vibration CH_2 rocking
Alkenes	3095–3075/3040–3010 1680–1600 2000–1900	med var str	=C—H and =CH_2 (usually sharp) C=C alkeyl, aryl, conjugated C=C asymmetric stretch	1420–1410/1310–1290 995–985/895–885 730–675 970–960	str med broad	=C—H and =CH_2 (in plane bend) =C—H and =CH_2 (out-of-plane bending) cis-RCH=CHR trans-RCH=CHR
Alkynes	3320–3310 2250–2100	str var	C—H (usually sharp) C≡C (symmetric reduces intensity)	680–610	str	C—H
Aromatic	3130–3070 1600–1500	var med-wk	C—H C=C (in ring) (2 bands) (3 if conjugated)	1225–950 900–670	str-med	C—H in-plane bend C—H out-of-plane bend
Alcohols & hydroxy	3645–3600 3645–3630 3635–3620 3620–3540/3640–3530 3570–3200 1200–1050	Var str str	O—H (free), usually sharp Primary O—H Secondary O—H Tertiary O—H/Phenols O—H O—H (H-bonded), usually broad C—O	1410–1310 720–560	med var-wk	O—H bending (in-plane) O—H bend (out-of-plane)
Amines	3400–3325 3510–3380 3360–3310 3490–3430 1090–1020/1190–1130 1210–1150	Wk wk med	N—H (1°-amines), 2 bands Aliphatic amines Aromatic amines N—H (2°-amines) Aliphatic amines Aromatic and heterocyclic amines C—N Primary/Secondary amines Tertiary amines	1650–1590 1650–1550 660–990	med-str var	N—H scissoring (1°-amines) =N—H (bend) NH_2 and N—H wagging (shifts on H-bonding)

	Stretching Vibrations			Bending Vibrations		
Functional Class	**Range (cm^{-1})**	**Intensity**	**Assignment**	**Range (cm^{-1})**	**Intensity**	**Assignment**
Aldehyde and ketones	2840–2690 (2 bands)	med	C—H (aldehyde C—H)	1360–1350	str	α-CH_3 bending
	1740–1720	str	C=O (saturated aldehyde)	1450–1400	str	α-CH_2 bending
	1720–1705	str	C=O (saturated ketone)	1100	med	C—C—C bending
	1820–1775	str	aryl carbonate	1360–1350	str	α-CH_3 bending
	1870–1790	str	Anhydride	1450–1400	str	α-CH_2 bending
	1680–1630	str	Amide	1100	med	C—C—C bending
	1750–1725	str	Easter			
Carboxylic acids and Derivatives	3300–2500 (acids)	str	O—H (very broad)	144–1390	med	C—O—H bending
	overlap C—H	str	C=O (H-bonded)			
	1720–1705 (acids)	med-str	O—C (sometimes 2-peaks)			
	1320–1210 (acids)					
	1815–1785 (acyl halides)	str	C=O			
	1870 and 1790 (anhydrides)	str	C=O (2-bands)			
	1100–1050					
	1750–1725 (esters)	str	O—C			
	1000–1300	str	C=O			
	1680–1630 (amides)	str	O—C (2-bands)	1650–1590	med	N—H (1-amide) II band
		str	C=O (amide I band)	1560–1500	med	N—H (2-amide) II band
Nitriles Isocyanates,	2280–2240	med	C≡N (sharp) Aliphatic cyanide	144–1390	med	C—O—H bending
	2240–2220	med	Aromatic cyanide			
Isothiocyanates, Diimides,	2276–2240		—N=C=O, Isocyanates			
Azides and Ketenes	2150–1990		—N=C=S, (Isotheonate)			
			—N=C=N—			
	1630–1575		—N_3 (open chain azo)			

OTHER FUNCTIONAL GROUPS

Infrared absorption data for some functional groups not listed in the preceding table are given below. Most of the absorptions cited are associated with stretching vibrations. Standard abbreviations (str = strong, wk = weak, brd = broad and shp = sharp) are used to describe the absorption bands.

Functional Class		Characteristic Absorptions
	Sulphur Functions	
S—H	thiols	2600–2550 cm^{-1} (wk & shp)
S—OR	esters	900–700 (str)
S—S	disulfide	620–600 (wk)
C=S	thiocarbonyl	1200–1050 (str)
S=O	sulfoxide sulfone sulfonic acid sulfonyl chloride sulfate	1060–1030 (str) 1325 ± 25 (as) & 1140 ± 20 (s) (both str) 1345 (str) 1365 ± 5 (as) & 1180 ± 10 (s) (both str) 1450–1350 (str)
	Phosphorous Functions	
P—H	phosphine	2440–2280 cm^{-1} (med and shp) 1250–950 (wk) P — H bending
(O=) PO—H	phosphoric acid	2700–2550 (med)
P—OR	esters	1050–990 (str)
P=O	phosphine oxide phosphonate phosphate phosphoramide	1200–1100 (str) 1260–1230 (str) 1200–1100 (str) 1275–1250 (str)
	Silicon Functions	
Si—H	silane	2360–2100 cm^{-1} (str)
Si—OR	1110–1080 (str and brd)	
Si—CH_3	1250 ± 10 (str and shp)	
	Oxidized Nitrogen Functions	
=NOH	oxime O—H (stretch) C=N N—O	3600–3550 cm^{-1} (str) 1665 ± 15945 ± 15
N—O	amine oxide aliphatic aromatic	960 ± 201250 ± 50
N=O	nitroso nitro	1550 ± 50 (str) 1530 ± 20 (as) and 1350 ± 30 (s)

A QUICK DIAGNOSTIC ASSESSMENT OF AN INFRARED SPECTRUM

When analysing an IR spectrum, avoid the temptation to try to assign every **peak.** The *fingerprint* region, however, can be useful for helping to confirm a structure by direct comparison with a known spectra.

Step 1: *Overall Spectrum Appearance*

If the spectrum is simple, compound may be a low-molecular-weight organic or inorganic compound, such as a simple salt of a common molecular ion (carbonate, sulphate, nitrate, ammonium, etc.) or a covalent species (chloroform, dichloromethane, methanol, water, etc.). One other class of compounds worth mentioning here is simple polymers, such as polyethylene and polytetrafluoroethylene, both of which exhibit very simple spectra when obtained from thin films.

If some of the bands are broad, hydrogen bonding possibly exists and can be exhibited in hydrates, water solutions, alcohols, ammonium compounds, amino compounds, etc. Note that some inorganics may exhibit a combination of both broad and very narrow bands, even for certain hydrated species.

Step 2: *Testing for Organics and Hydrocarbons — Absorptions in the Region 3200–2700 cm*$^{-1}$

Well-defined and characteristic absorptions in this region are normally characteristic of C—H containing species, and are assigned to various forms of C—H stretching.

If the absorptions above 3000 cm^{-1}, compound is likely to be unsaturated (contains C=C) or aromatic. If isolated absorptions occur at 3010 and/or 3040 cm^{-1}, then the absorbing species is mostly simple olefinic unsaturation.

Is the main absorption below 3000 cm^{-1}, compound is probably aliphatic. If the main absorptions are approximately 2935 and 2860 cm^{-1}, and there are also absorptions at 1470 and 720 cm^{-1}, then the compound probably contains a long linear aliphatic chain.

Step 3: *Testing for Hydroxy or Amino Groups — Absorptions in the Region 3650–3250 cm*$^{-1}$

Hydroxy or amino groups mainly dominate this region, both giving rise to very characteristic band profiles. If the main absorption band in the area broad, compound is probably a hydroxy or amino group. If there additional moderate to intense bands in the ranges 1600–1300, 1200–1000 and 800–600 cm^{-1}.

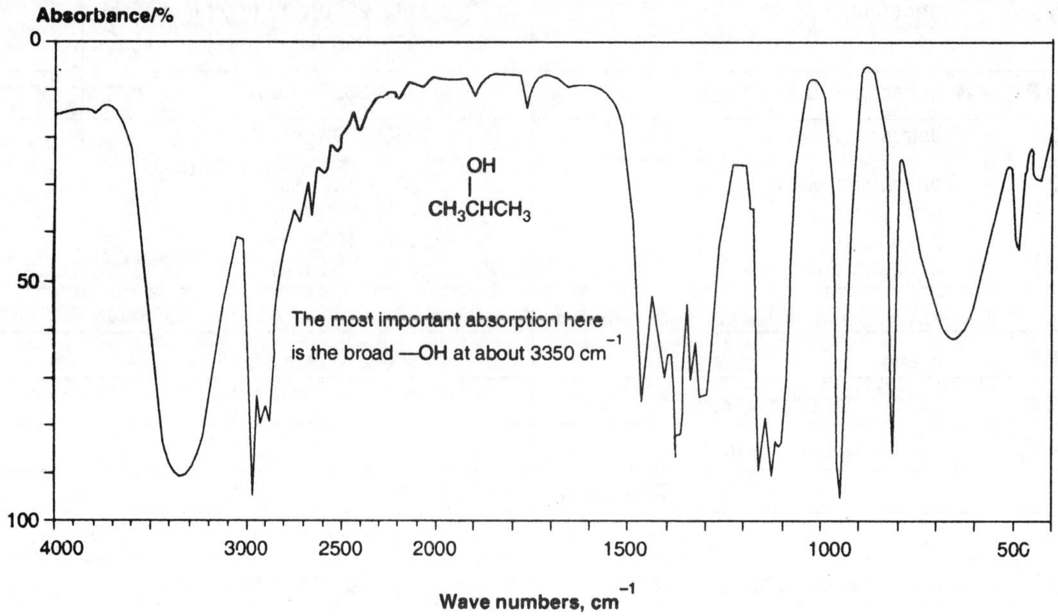

Step 4: *Testing for Carbonyl Compounds — Absorptions in the Region 1850–1650 cm*$^{-1}$

If the absorption at the high end of the range, e.g. 1775 cm^{-1} or above, compound probably contains a reactive carbonyl, such as an anhydride, acid halide (acyl halide) or a-halogenated carbonyl or a strained-ring carbonyl, such as a lactone or an organic carbonate.

If the absorption in the middle of the range is 1750–1700 cm^{-1}, compound is probably a simple carbonyl compound, such as a ketone, an aldehyde, an ester, or a carboxylic acid.

If the absorption at the low end of the range, e.g. below 1700 cm^{-1}, compound is probably an amide or a carboxylate (carboxylic acid salt). Note that conjugation with another carbonyl group, or a double bond or aromatic ring, will lower the carbonyl absorption by 30–50 cm^{-1}.

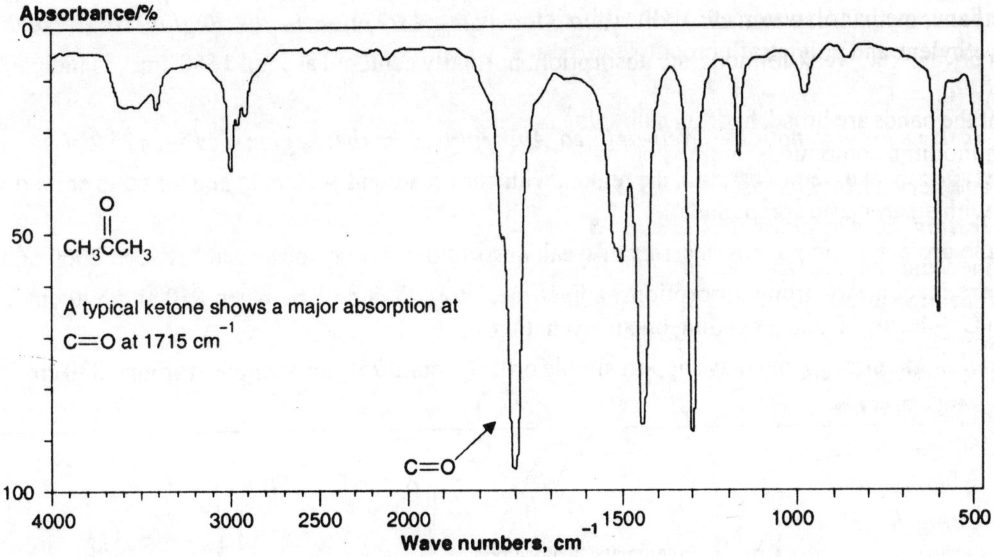
Absorbance/%
0
50
100
CH3CCH3 (O above the central C)
A typical ketone shows a major absorption at
C=O at 1715 cm-1
C=O
4000
3000
2500
2000
1500
1000
500
Wave numbers, cm-1

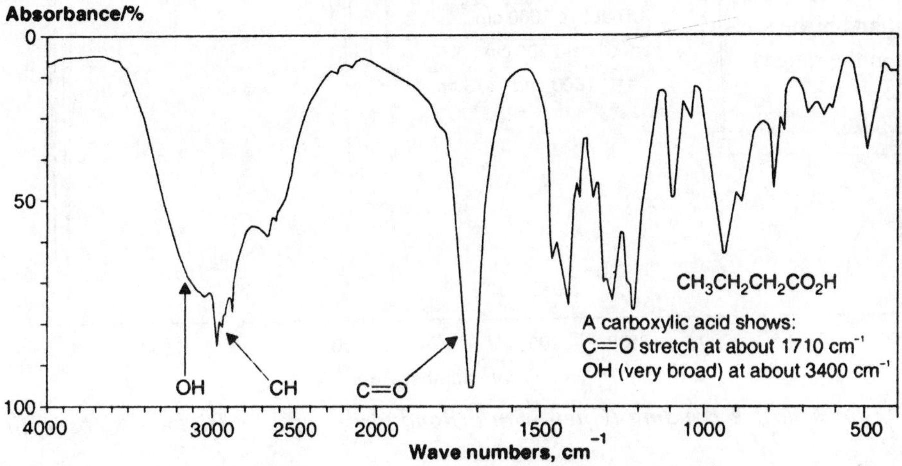
Absorbance/%
0
50
100
CH3CH2CH2CO2H
A carboxylic acid shows:
C=O stretch at about 1710 cm-1
OH (very broad) at about 3400 cm-1
OH
CH
C=O
4000
3000
2500
2000
1500
1000
500
Wave numbers, cm-1

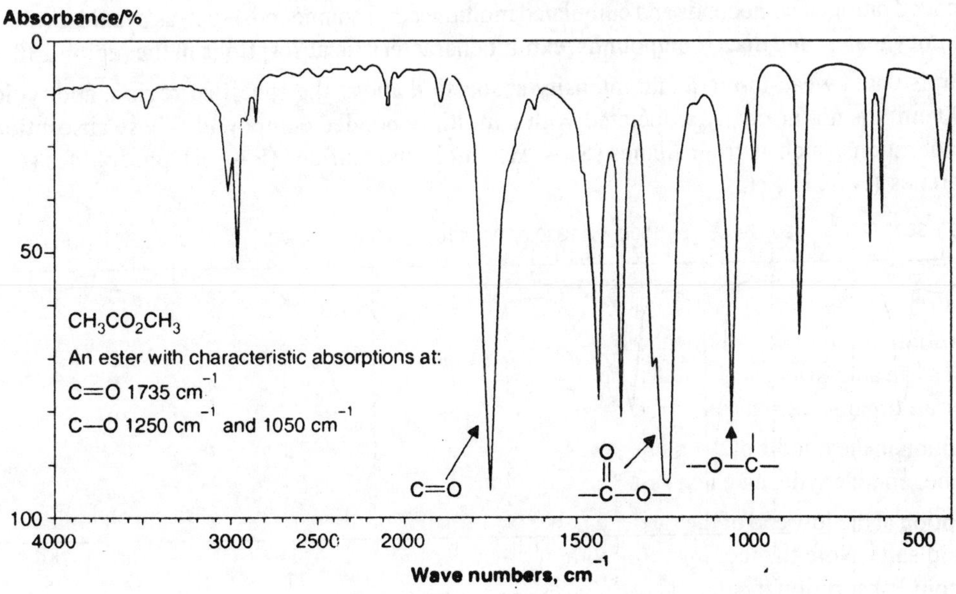
Absorbance/%
0
50
100
CH3CO2CH3
An ester with characteristic absorptions at:
C=O 1735 cm-1
C—O 1250 cm-1 and 1050 cm-1
C=O
—C—O— (O above the C)
—O—C—
4000
3000
2500
2000
1500
1000
500
Wave numbers, cm-1

Step 5: Testing for Unsaturation — Weak to Moderate Absorption in the Region 1670–1620 cm⁻¹

A relatively narrow, weak-to-moderate absorption, normally centered around 1650 cm^{-1}, is indicative of olefinic unsaturation (C = C).

Step 6: Testing for Aromatics — Well-defined Absorptions in the Region 1615–1495 cm⁻¹

One, but typically two, sets of bands in the region, with one set around 1600 cm^{-1} and the other around 1500 cm^{-1}, are consistent with an aromatic compound.

For simple aromatic compounds, a series of weak absorptions may be observed between 2000 and 1700 cm^{-1}.

If there are medium-to-strong absorptions, sometimes more than one, between 850 and 670 cm^{-1}, these can be assigned to C—H out-of-plane bending on an aromatic ring.

Note that a single, strong band may support simple ortho (around 750 cm^{-1}) or para (around 830 cm^{-1}) substitution.

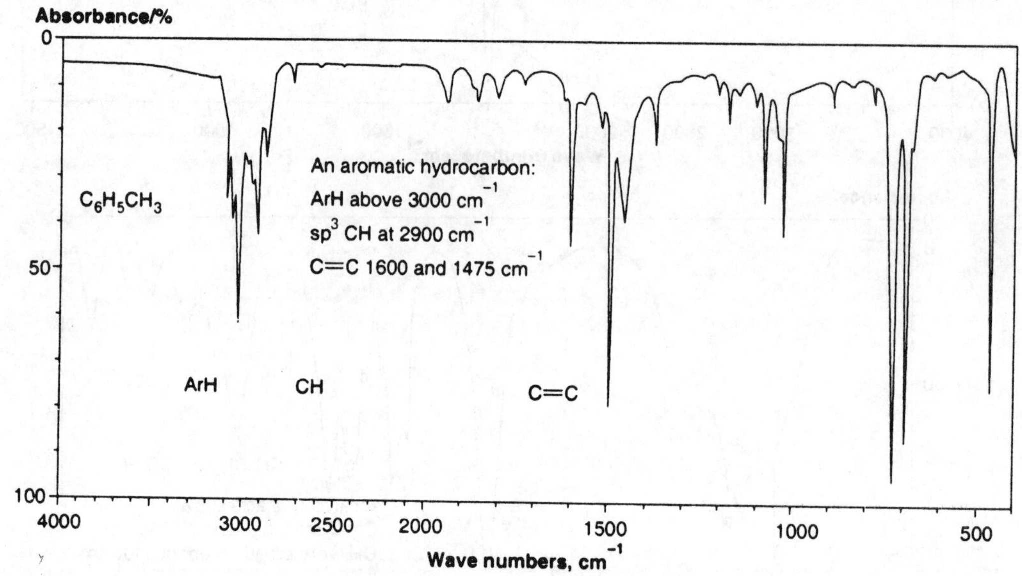

Step 7: Testing for Multiple Bonding (Often with a Bond Order of 2 or Higher) – Absorption in the Region 2300–1990 cm⁻¹

Multiply bonded nitrogen compounds and cumulated multiple bond compounds, such as cyanides (nitriles), cyanates, isocyanates, thiocyanates, and diazo compounds, exhibit characteristic absorptions in the region 2300–1990 cm^{-1}.

Note that an isolated weak-to-moderate intensity absorption above the specified region, and typically between 2700 and 2400 cm^{-1}, is not normally associated with a multiply bonded compound. These absorptions are usually from hydride vibrations, such as from silanes (Si — H), thiols and sulfides (S — H), phosphines (P — H), arsines (As — H), boranes (B — H), etc.

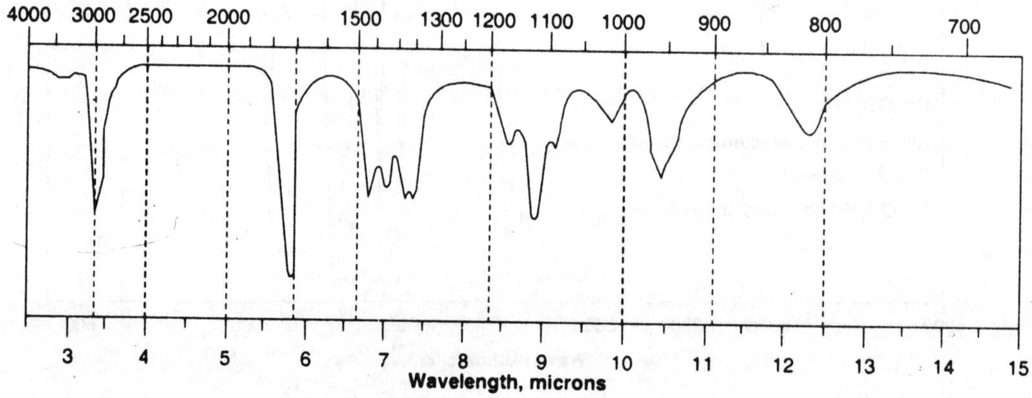

$C_5H_{10}O$

From the molecular formula, the compound has "1 degree of unsaturation" (one double bond, carbonyl or ring).

3400–3200 cm^{-1} : no OH or NH present

3100 cm^{-1} : no peak to suggest unsaturated CH

2900 cm^{-1} : strong peak indicating saturated CH

2200 cm^{-1} : no unsymmetrical triple bonds

1710 cm^{-1} : strong carbonyl absorbance

1610 cm^{-1} : no absorbance to suggest carbon-carbon double bonds

The spectrum seems to be consistent with a simple aliphatic carbonyl compound.

Structure

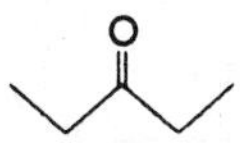

IUPAC Name: 3-pentanone (diethyl ketone)

Analysis-2: C_8H_8O

IR Spectrum

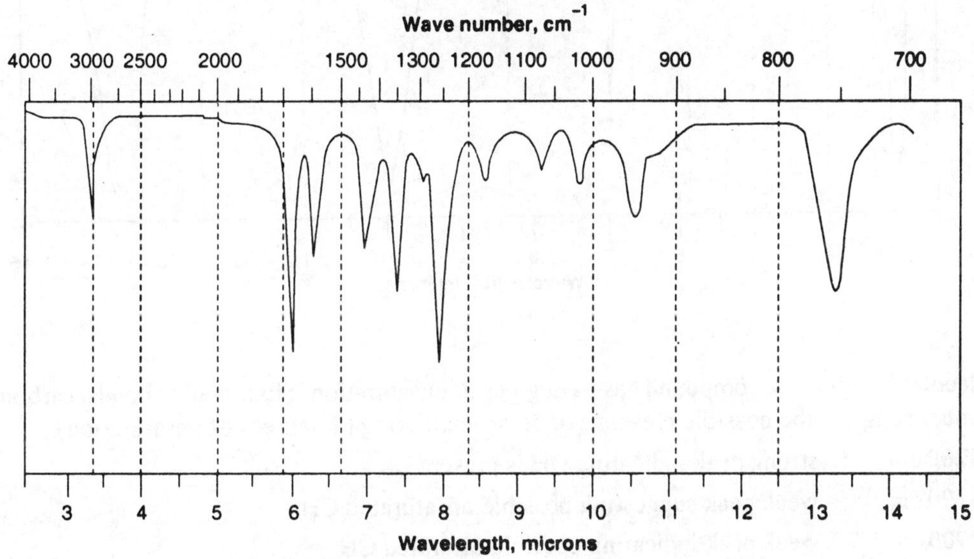

C_8H_8O

From the molecular formula, the compound has "5 degrees of unsaturation" (five double bonds, carbonyls or rings). The large number suggests the possible presence of an aromatic ring (4 degrees of unsaturation).

3400–3200 cm^{-1} : no OH or NH present

3100 cm^{-1} : moderate peak suggesting unsaturated CH

2900 cm^{-1} : weak peak indicating possible saturated CH

2200 cm^{-1} : no unsymmetrical triple bonds

1690 cm^{-1} : strong carbonyl absorbance

1610 cm^{-1} : weak absorbance bands consistent with carbon-carbon double bonds

The spectrum seems to be consistent with a carbonyl compound containing both single and double bonds. The carbonyl absorbance occurs at a relatively low wave number, suggesting the carbonyl is conjugated with a double bond or an aromatic ring. The large number of degrees of unsaturation suggests the presence of an aromatic ring.

Structure

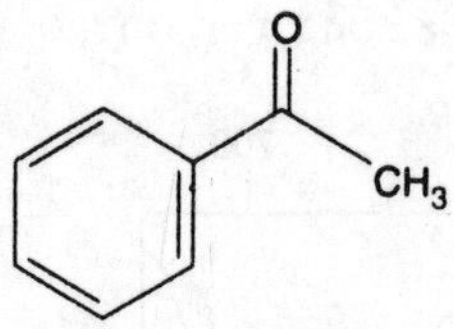

IUPAC Name: acetophenone

Analysis-3: C_7H_8O
IR Spectrum

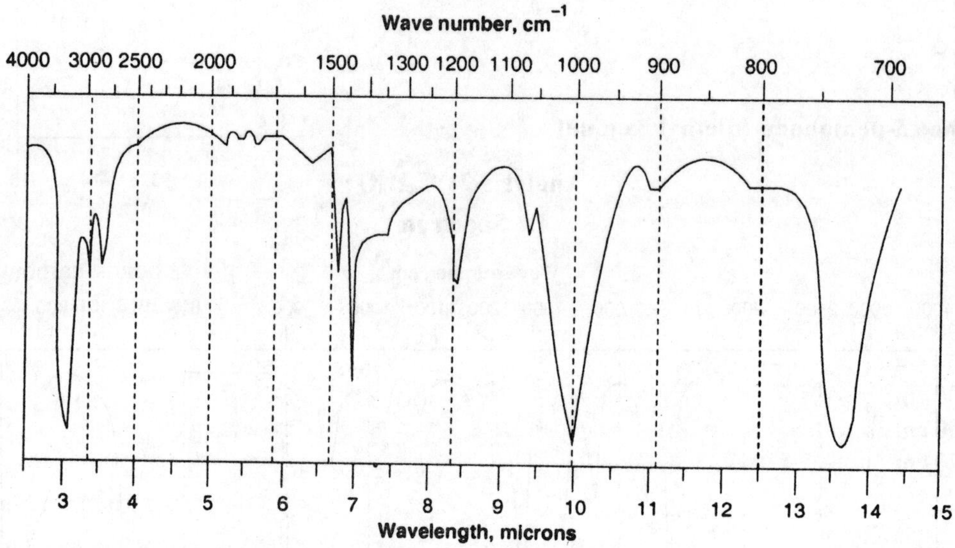

C_7H_8O

From the molecular formula, the compound has "4 degrees of unsaturation" (four double bonds, carbonyls or rings). The large number suggests the possible presence of an aromatic ring (4 degrees of unsaturation).

3400–3200 cm^{-1}	:	strong peak indicating OH is present
3100 cm^{-1}	:	weak peak suggesting possible unsaturated CH
2900 cm^{-1}	:	weak peak indicating possible saturated CH
2200 cm^{-1}	:	no unsymmetrical triple bonds
1720 cm^{-1}	:	no carbonyl absorbance
1450–1500 cm^{-1}	:	moderate absorbance bands consistent with aromatic carbon-carbon double bonds

The spectrum seems to be consistent with an alcohol containing both single and double bonds. The large number of degrees of unsaturation suggests the presence of an aromatic ring.

Structure

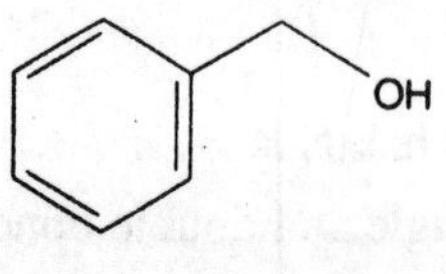

IUPAC Name: benzyl alcohol

Analysis-4: C_8H_7N
IR Spectrum

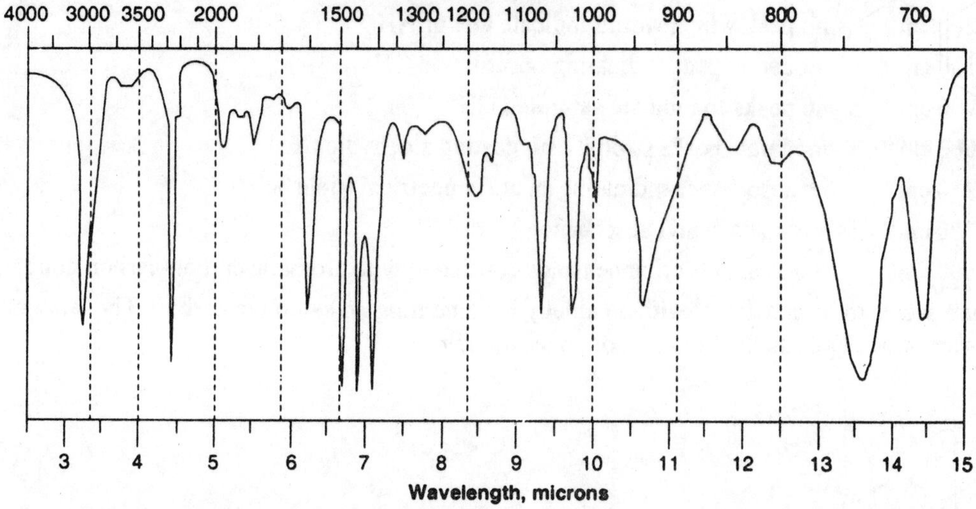

C_8H_7N

From the molecular formula, the compound has "6 degrees of unsaturation" (six double bonds, carbonyls or rings). The large number suggests the possible presence of an aromatic ring (4 degrees of unsaturation).

3400–3200 cm^{-1}	:	no peak which would indicate OH or NH
3100 cm^{-1}	:	strong peak suggesting unsaturated CH
2900 cm^{-1}	:	moderate peak indicating saturated CH
2250 cm^{-1}	:	strong absorbance indicating an unsymmetrical triple bond
1720 cm^{-1}	:	no carbonyl absorbance
1450–1600 cm^{-1}	:	moderate absorbance bands consistent with aromatic carbon-carbon double bonds

The spectrum seems to be consistent with a nitrile (—C≡N) containing both single and double bonds. The large number of degrees of unsaturation suggests the presence of an aromatic ring.

Structure

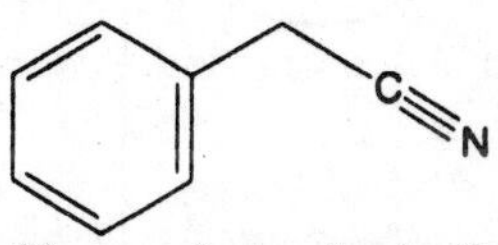

IUPAC Name: benzyl nitrile

Analysis-5: C_7H_6O
IR Spectrum

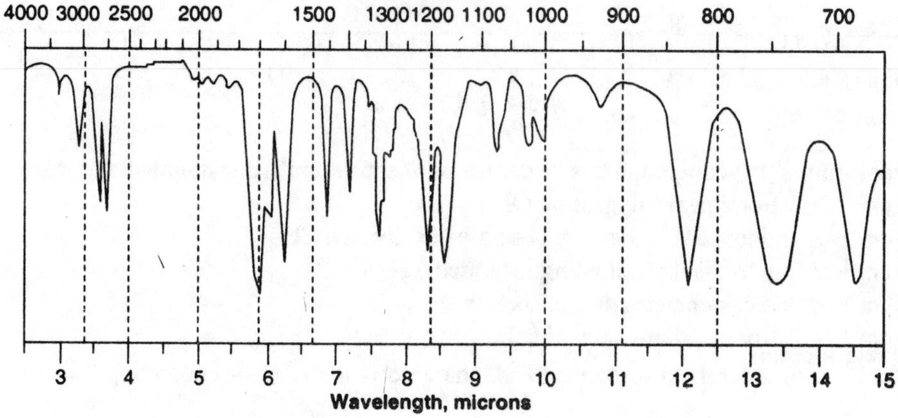

C_7H_6O

From the molecular formula, the compound has "5 degrees of unsaturation" (five double bonds, carbonyls or rings). The large number suggests the possible presence of an aromatic ring (4 degrees of unsaturation).

3400–3200 cm^{-1} : no peak which would indicate OH or NH
3100 cm^{-1} : moderate peak indicating unsaturated CH
2900 cm^{-1} : no peaks to indicate saturated CH
2750–2600 cm^{-1} : moderate peaks strongly suggesting aldehydic CH
2250 cm^{-1} : no absorbance indicating an unsymmetrical triple bonds
1700 cm^{-1} : strong carbonyl absorbance
1450–1600 cm^{-1} : moderate absorbance bands consistent with aromatic carbon-carbon double bonds

The spectrum seems to be consistent with an aldehyde containing no saturated carbon. The large number of degrees of unsaturation suggests the presence of an aromatic ring.

Structure

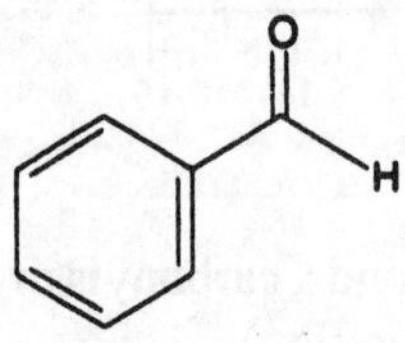

IUPAC Name: benzaldehyde

Analysis-6: $C_3H_{10}NO$
IR Spectrum

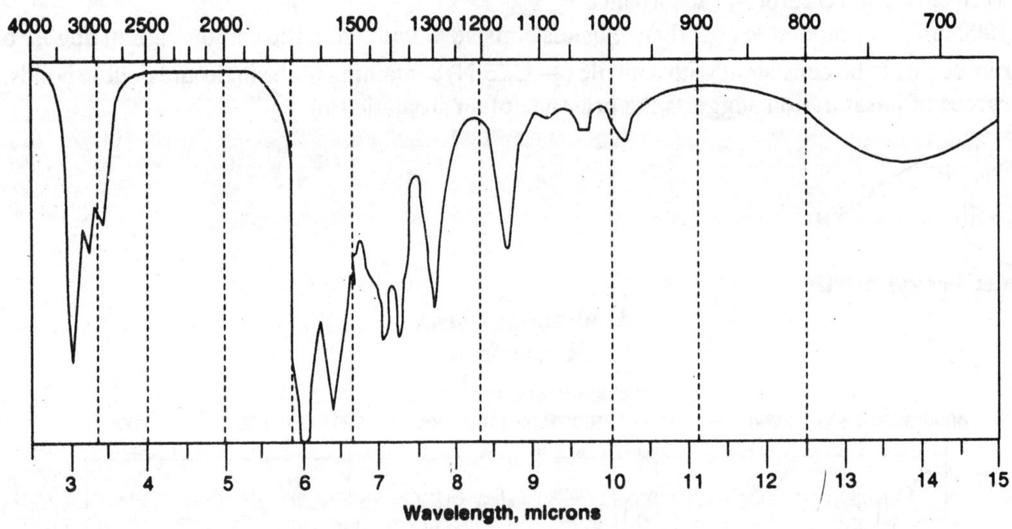

$C_3H_{10}NO$

From the molecular formula, the compound has "1 degree of unsaturation" (one double bond, carbonyl or ring).

3400–3200 cm^{-1} : strong peak suggesting OH or NH
3100 cm^{-1} : minor peak indicating possible unsaturated CH
2900 cm^{-1} : minor peaks indicating saturated CH
2200 cm^{-1} : no unsymmetrical triple bonds
1650 cm^{-1} : strong carbonyl absorbance
1550 cm^{-1} : moderate absorbance band, characteristic of "N — H bending"

The spectrum seems to be consistent with a compound containing a carbonyl group and an N—H group. The low carbonyl band (1650 cm^{-1}) and the N—H bending band strongly suggest an amide linkage; this pair of absorbance are often termed the "amide I and II" bands.

Structure

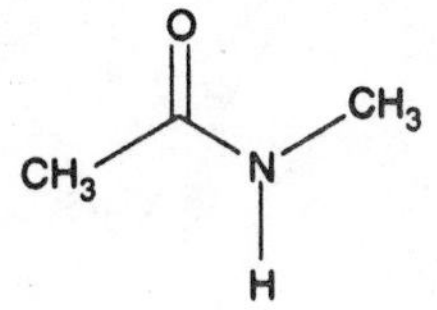

IUPAC Name: N-methylacetamide (N-methylethanamide)

Analysis-7: $C_4H_8O_2$
IR Spectrum

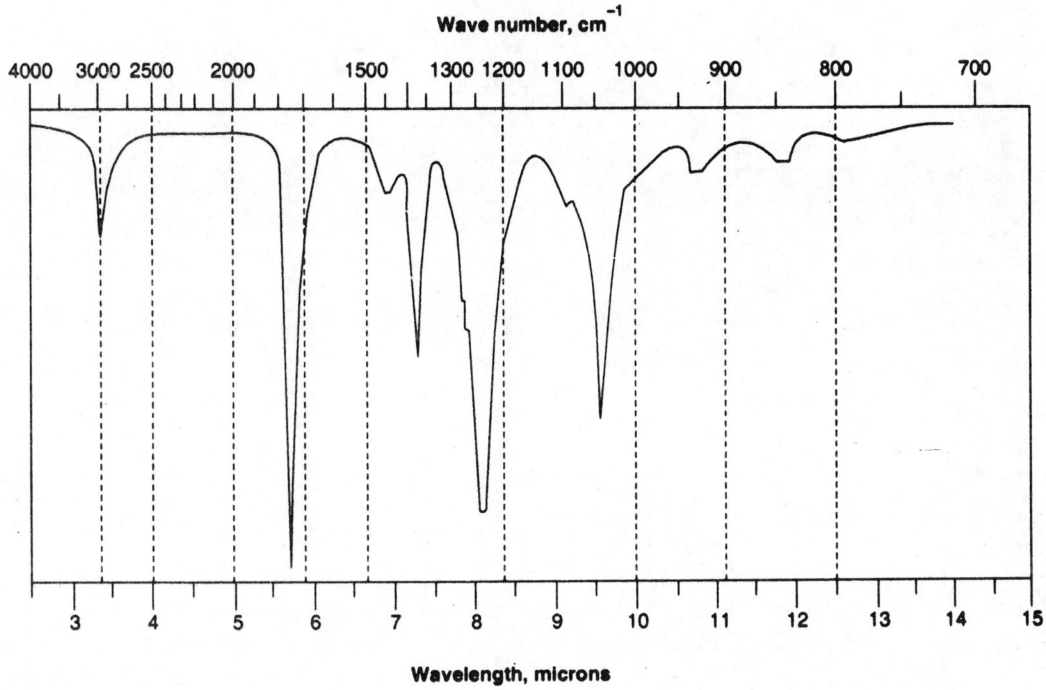

$C_4H_8O_2$

From the molecular formula, the compound has "1 degree of unsaturation" (one double bond, carbonyl or ring).

3400–3200 cm^{-1} : no peak to indicate an OH or NH
3100 cm^{-1} : no peak to indicate unsaturated CH
2900 cm^{-1} : minor peaks indicating saturated CH
2200 cm^{-1} : no unsymmetrical triple bonds
1760 cm^{-1} : strong carbonyl absorbance
1600 cm^{-1} : no peak to indicate a carbon-carbon double bond
1250 cm^{-1} : strong, broad peak consistent with a carbon-oxygen single bond

The spectrum seems to be consistent with a compound containing a carbonyl group and only saturated C — H. The carbonyl band is relatively high (1760 cm^{-1}) suggestive of an ester linkage. The band at 1250 cm is consistent with a CO bond, but many things absorb in this region.

Structure

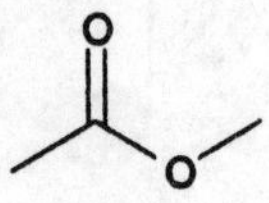

IUPAC Name: ethyl acetate (ethyl ethanoate)

Mass Spectroscopy

11

INTRODUCTION

Mass spectrometry has become one of the most important analytical tools of today. The use of it has spread to a large number of areas such as molecular physics, chemistry, biology and medicine. The very first study of positive rays was due to J.J. Thomson who gave a detailed account of it in his "Rays of Positive Electricity and their Application to Chemical Analysis". New methods of ion production, novel tools for desorption, methods of mass analysis, detection and data manipulation have made it possible to analyze almost anything by mass spectrometry. Mass limits are being stretched and sensitivity limits are broken routinely. Along with these advances in instrumentation, altogether new chemistry of ions is being explored.

Mass spectrometry is based on slightly different principles to the other spectroscopic methods.

The physics behind mass spectrometry is that a charged particle passing through a magnetic field is deflected along a circular path on a radius that is proportional to the mass to charge ratio, m/e. In an electron impact mass spectrometer, a high-energy beam of electrons is used to displace an electron from the organic molecule to form a *radical cation* known as the *molecular ion*. If the molecular ion is too unstable then it can *fragment* to give other smaller ions.

The collection of ions is then focused into a beam and accelerated into the magnetic field and deflected along circular paths according to the masses of the ions. By adjusting the magnetic field, the ions can be focused on the detector and recorded.

In an electron impact mass spectrometer, a high-energy beam of electrons is used to displace an electron from the organic molecule to form a *radical cation* known as the *molecular ion*. If the molecular ion is too unstable, then it can *fragment* to give other smaller ions. The collection of ions is then focused into a beam and accelerated into the magnetic field and deflected along circular paths according to the masses of the ions. By adjusting the magnetic field, the ions can be focused on the detector and recorded

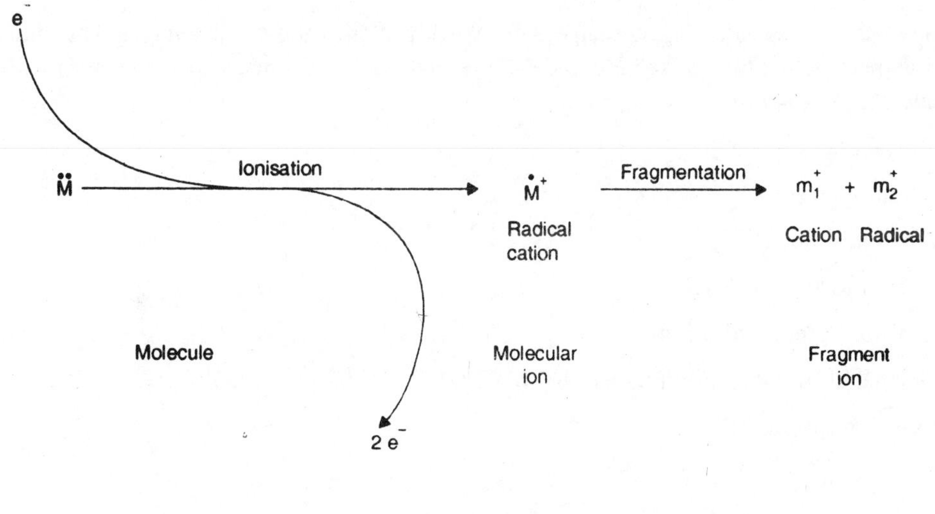

Terminology

Molecular ion	The ion obtained by the loss of an electron from the molecule
Base peak	The most intense peak in the MS, assigned 100% intensity
M^{+}	Symbol often given to the molecular ion
Radical cation	+ve charged species with an odd number of electrons
Fragment ions	Lighter cations formed by the decomposition of the molecular ion. These often correspond to stable carbcations.

Sample Introduction

The method of sample introduction to the ionisation source often depends on the ionisation method being used, as well as the type and complexity of the sample. The sample can be inserted directly into the ionisation source, or can undergo some type of chromatography *en route* to the ionisation source. This latter method of sample introduction usually involves the mass spectrometer being coupled directly to a high pressure liquid chromatography (HPLC), gas chromatography (GC) or capillary electrophoresis (CE) separation column, and hence the sample is separated into a series of components which then enter the mass spectrometer sequentially for individual analysis.

- For large samples such as **biomolecules,** molecular masses can be measured to within an accuracy of **0.01%** of the total molecular mass of the sample, *i.e.* within a 4 Daltons (Da) or atomic mass units (amu) error for a sample of 40,000 Da. This is sufficient to allow minor mass changes to be detected, *e.g.* the substitution of one amino acid for another, or a post-translational modification.

For small **organic molecules** the molecular mass can be measured to within an accuracy of **5 ppm** or less, which is often sufficient to confirm the molecular formula of a compound, and is also a standard requirement for publication in a chemical journal.

Structural information can be generated using certain types of mass spectrometers, usually those with multiple analysers which are known as **tandem mass spectrometers.** This is achieved by fragmenting the sample inside the instrument and analysing the products generated. This procedure is useful for the structural elucidation of **organic compounds** and for **peptide** or **oligonucleotide** sequence.

Methods of Sample Ionisation

Many ionisation methods are available and each has its own advantages and disadvantages. The ionisation method to be used should depend on the type of sample under investigation and the mass spectrometer available. *Ionisation methods include the following:*

1. Electron Impact (EI)
2. Chemical Ionisation (CI)
3. Electrospray Ionisation (ESI)
4. Fast Atom Bombardment (FAB)
5. Field Desorption / Field Ionisation (FD/FI)
6. Matrix Assisted Laser Desorption Ionisation (MALDI)
7. Thermospray Ionisation (TSP)

Table: Summarize table of some important ionization method with specific properties.

Ionization method	Typical analytes	Sample introduction	Mass range	Method highlights
Electron Impact (EI)	Relatively small volatile	GC or liquid/solid probe	to 1,000 Daltons	Hard method versatile provides structure info
Chemical Ionization (CI)	Relatively small volatile	GC or liquid/solid probe	to 1,000 Daltons	Soft method molecular ion peak $[M + H]^+$
Electro spray (ESI)	Peptides, Proteins and Nonvolatiles	Liquid chromatography or syringe	to 200,000 Daltons	Soft method ions often multiply charged
Fast Atom Bombardment (FAB)	Carbohydrates Organometallics Peptides Nonvolatile	Sample mixed in viscous matrix	to 6,000 Daltons	Soft method but harder than ESI or MALDI
Matrix Assisted Laser Desorption Ionisation (MALDI)	Peptides Proteins Nucleotides	Sample mixed matrix	to 500,000 Daltons	Soft method very high mass

Analysis and Separation of Sample Ions

Several forms of mass analyzer which separate ions according to their mass-to-charge ratio exits, e.g. magnetic sector analyzers, quadrupole mass filters, time of flight analyzers, and ion cyclotron resonance instruments. The first two types, which account for the great majority of instruments used in organic analysis.

Table: Summarize types of analyzer used in mass spectrometer.

Analyzer	System highlights
Quadrupole	Unit mass resolution, fast scan, low cost
Sector (Magnetic and/or Electrostatic)	High resolution, exact mass
Time-of-Flight (TOF)	Theoretically, no limitation for m/z maximum, high throughput
Ion Cyclotron Resonance (IÇR)	Very high resolution, exact mass, perform ion chemistry

Isotopes: Isotopes occur in compounds analyzed by mass spectrometry in the same abundances that they occur in nature. A few of the isotopes commonly encountered in the analyses of organic compounds are below along with an example of how they can aid in peak identification.

Relative Isotope Abundance of Common Elements

Element	Isotope	Relative abundance	Isotope	Relative abundance	Isotope	Relative abundance
Carbon	^{12}C	100	^{13}C	1.11		
Hydrogen	^{1}H	100	^{2}H	.016		
Nitrogen	^{14}N	100	^{15}N	.38		
Oxygen	^{16}O	100	^{17}O	.04	^{18}O	.20
Sulfur	^{32}S	100	^{33}S	.78	^{34}S	4.40
Chlorine	^{35}Cl	100			^{37}Cl	32.5
Bromine	^{79}Br	100			^{81}Br	98.0

The following two mass spectra show examples of haloalkanes with characteristic isotope patterns.

Sample-01, 2-chloropropane

Note the isotope pattern at 78 and 80 that represent the *M* and *M* + 2 in a 3:1 ratio. Loss of ^{35}Cl from 78 or ^{37}Cl from 80 gives the base peak a m/z = 43, corresponding to the secondary propyl cation. Note that the peaks at m/z = 63 and 65 still contain Cl and therefore also show the 3:1 isotope pattern.

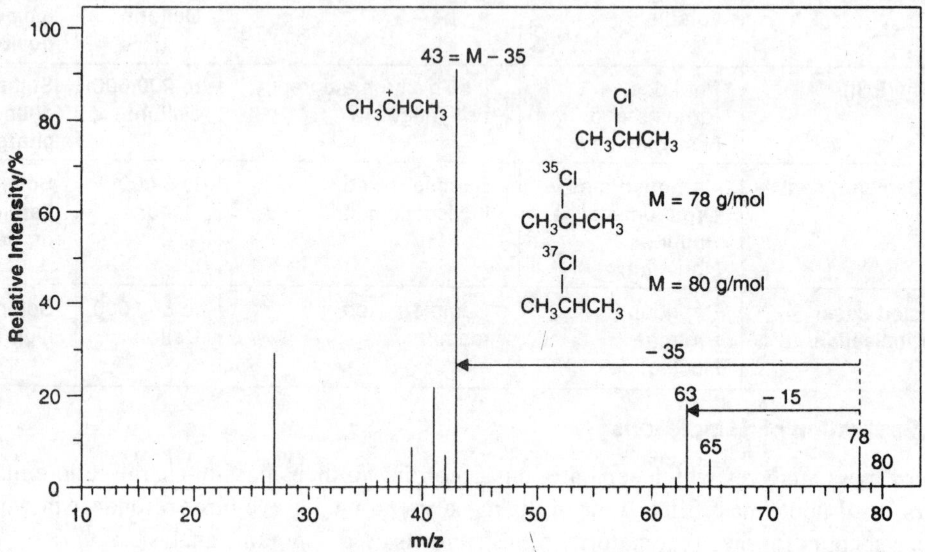

Sample-02, 1-bromopropane

Note the isotope pattern at 122 and 124 that represent the *M* and *M* + 2 in a 1:1 ratio. Loss of ^{79}Br from 122 or ^{81}Br from 124 gives the base peak a m/z = 43, corresponding to the propyl cation. Note that other peaks, such as those at m/z = 107 and 109 still contain Br and therefore also show the 1:1 isotope pattern.

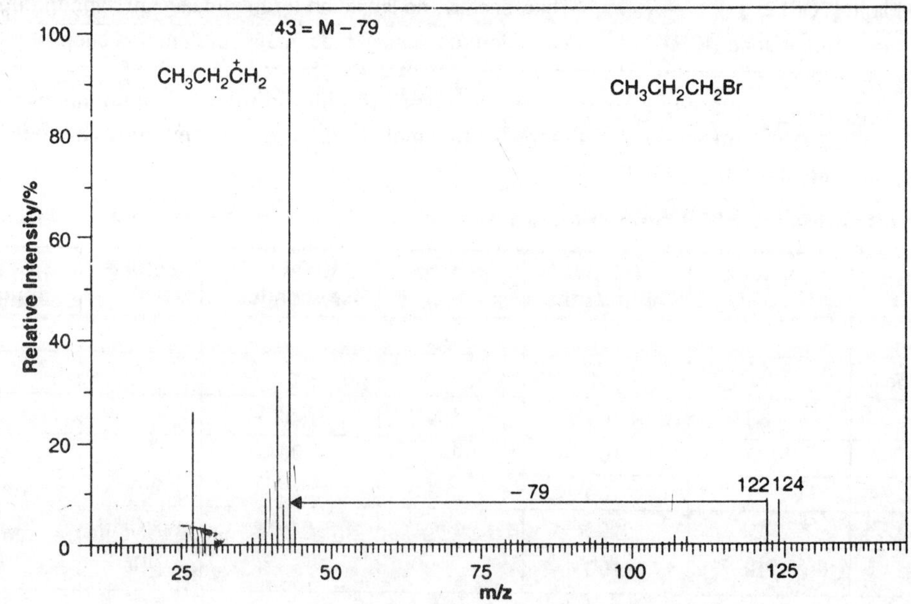

Detection and Recording of Sample Ions

The **detector** monitors the ion current, amplifies it and the signal is then transmitted to the data system where it is recorded in the form of **mass spectra**. The **m/z** values of the ions are plotted against their **intensities** to show the **number of components** in the sample, the **molecular mass** of each component, and the **relative abundance** of the various components in the sample. The type of detector is supplied to suit the type of analyser; the more common ones are the **photomultiplier,** the **electron multiplier** and the **micro-channel plate** detectors.

Steps to Interpret a Mass Spectrum

1. **Look for the molecular ion peak**
   - This peak (if it appears) will be the highest mass peak in the spectrum, except for isotope peaks.
   - Nominal MW (meaning=rounded off) will be an even number for compounds containing only C, H, O, S, Si.
   - Nominal MW will be an odd number if the compound also contains an odd number of N (1, 3,...).

2. **Try to calculate the molecular formula**
   - The isotope peaks can be very useful, and are best explained with an example.
     - Carbon-12 has an isotope, carbon-13. Their abundances are $^{12}C = 100\%$, $^{13}C = 1.1\%$. This means that for every 100 ^{12}C atoms there are 1.1 ^{13}C atoms.
     - If a compound contains 6 carbons, then each atom has a 1.1% abundance of ^{13}C.
     - Therefore, if the molecular ion peak is 100%, then the isotope peak (1 mass unit higher) would be $6 \times 1.1\% = 6.6\%$.
     - If the molecular ion peak is not 100%, then you can calculate the relative abundance of the isotope peak to the ion peak. For example, if the molecular ion peak were 34% and the isotope peak 2.3%: $(2.3/34) \times 100 = 6.8\%$. 6.8% is the relative abundance of the isotope peak to the ion peak. Next, divide the relative abundance by the isotope abundance: $6.8/1.1 = 6$ carbons.
   - Follow this order when looking for information provided by isotopes: (A simplified table of isotopes is provided in the introduction, more detailed tables can be found in chemistry texts.)
     - Look for A+2 elements: O, Si, S, Cl, Br
     - Look for A+1 elements: C, N
     - "A" elements: H, F, P, I

3. **Calculate the total number of rings plus double bonds**
   - For the molecular formula: $C_xH_yN_zO_n$
     - rings + double bonds $= x - (1/2)y + (1/2)z + 1$

4. **Postulate the molecular structure consistent with abundance and m/z of fragments**

   Following are examples of compounds listed by functional group, which demonstrate patterns which can be seen in mass spectra of compounds ionized by electron impact ionization. These examples do not provide information about the fragmentation mechanisms that cause these patterns.

ALCOHOL

An alcohol's molecular ion is small or non-existent. Cleavage of the C—C bond next to the oxygen usually occurs. A loss of H_2O may occur as in the spectra given:

3-Pentanol $C_5H_{12}O$ MW = 88.15

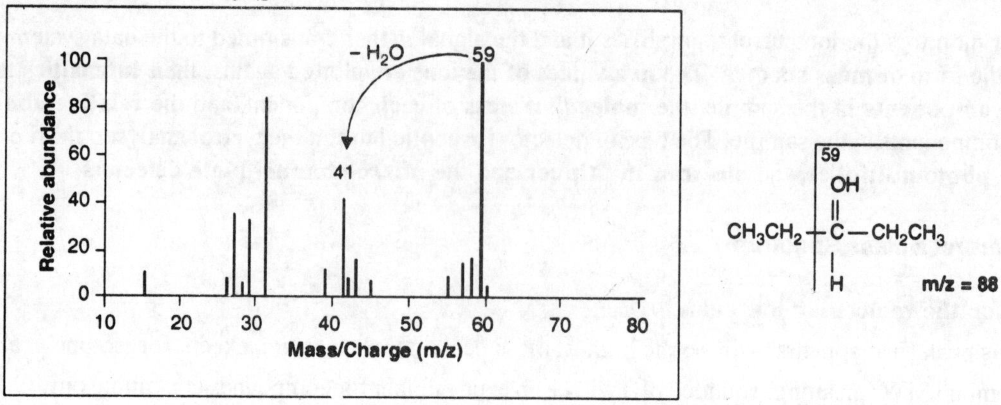

ALDEHYDE

Cleavage of bonds next to the carboxyl group results in the loss of hydrogen (molecular ion less 1) or the loss of CHO (molecular ion less 29).

3-Phenyl-2-propenal C_9H_8O MW = 132.16

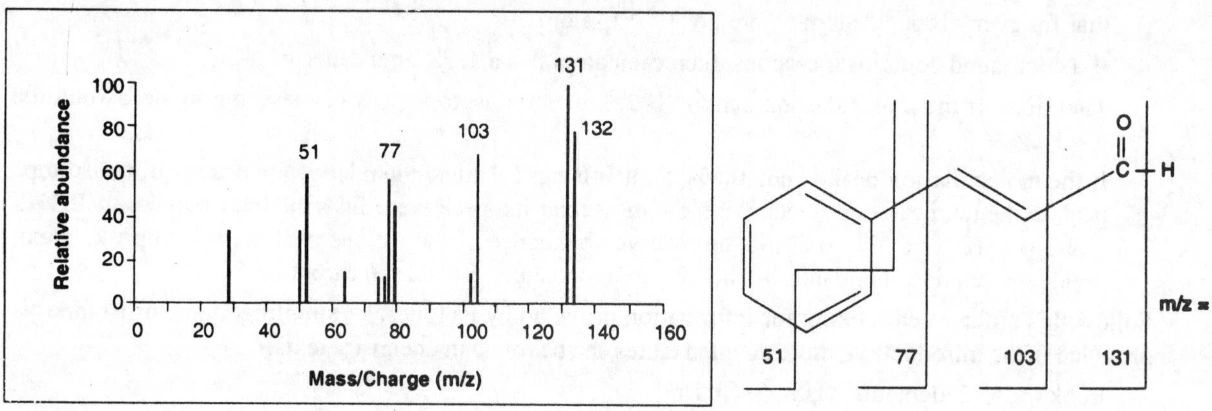

ALKANE

Molecular ion peaks are present, possibly with low intensity. The fragmentation pattern contains clusters of peaks 14 mass units apart (which represent loss of $(CH_2)_nCH_3$).

Hexane C_6H_{14} MW = 86.18

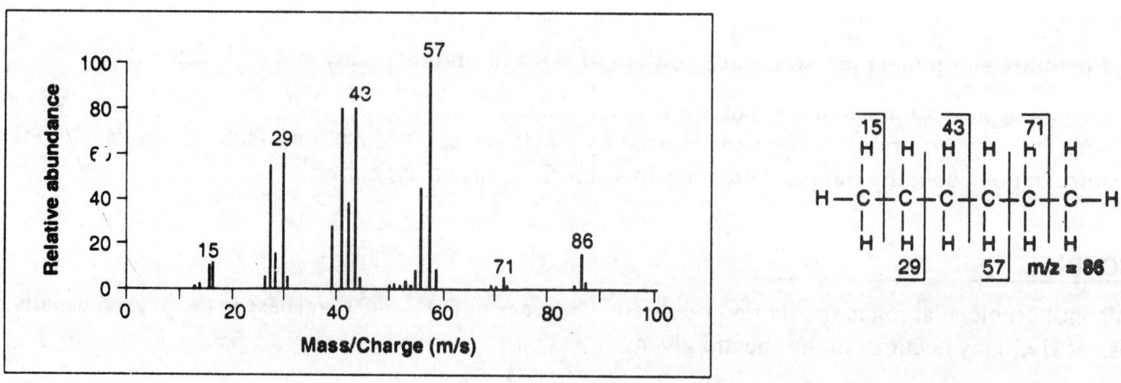

AMIDE

Primary amides show a base peak due to the McLafferty rearrangement.

3-Methylbutyramide $C_5H_{11}NO$ **MW = 101.15**

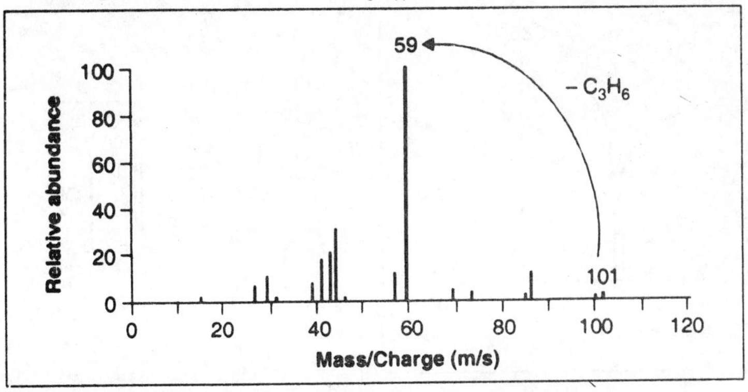

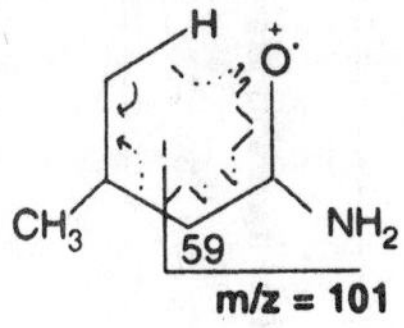

AMINE

Molecular ion peak is an odd number. Alpha-cleavage dominates aliphatic amines.

n-Butylamine $C_4H_{11}N$ **MW = 73.13**

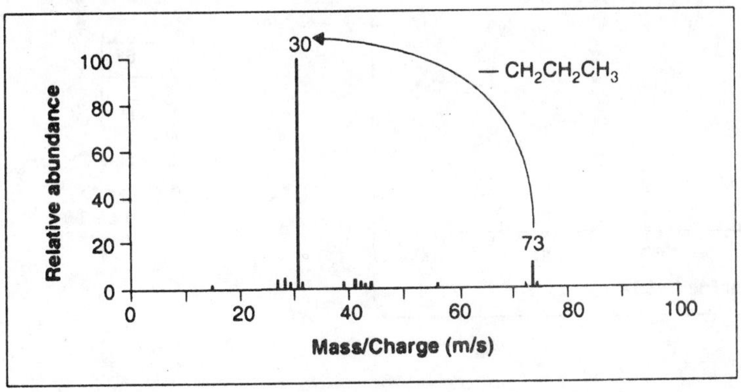

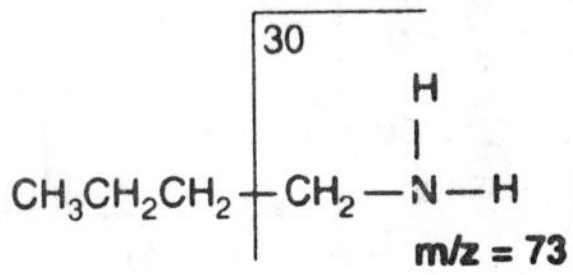

AROMATIC

Molecular ion peaks are strong due to the stable structure.

Naphthalene $C_{10}H_8$ **MW = 128.17**

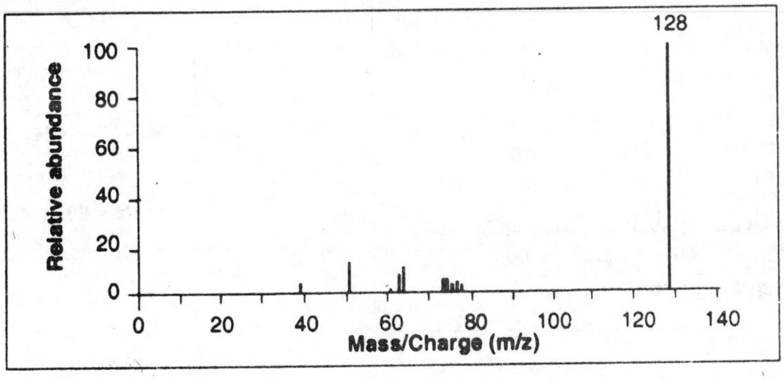

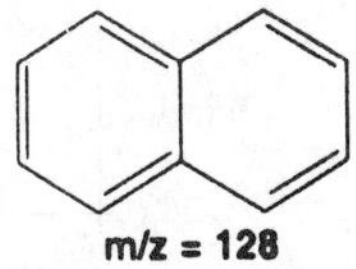

m/z = 128

CARBOXYLIC ACID

In short chain acids, peaks due to the loss of OH (molecular ion less 17) and COOH (molecular ion less 45) are prominent due to cleavage of bonds next to C=O.

2-Butenoic acid $C_4H_6O_2$ **MW = 86.09**

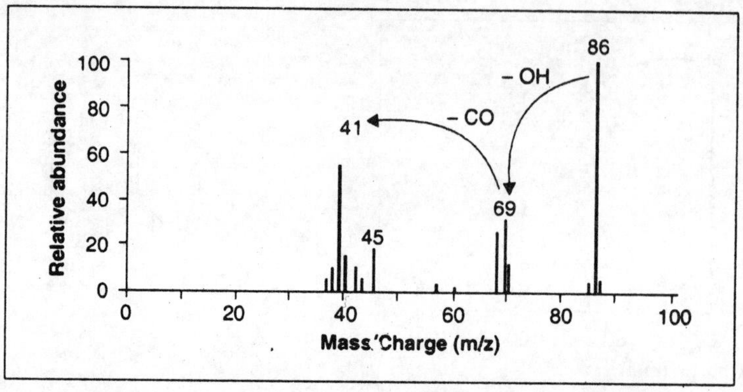

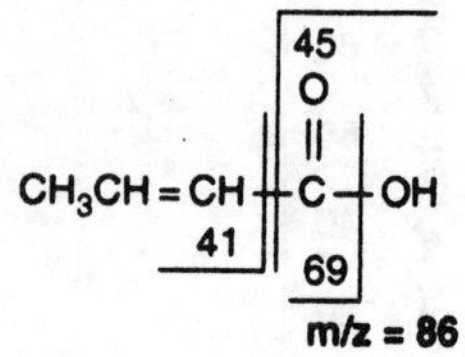

ESTER

Fragments appear due to bond cleavage next to C=O (alkoxy group loss, —OR) and hydrogen rearrangements.

Ethyl acetate $C_4H_8O_2$ **MW = 88.11**

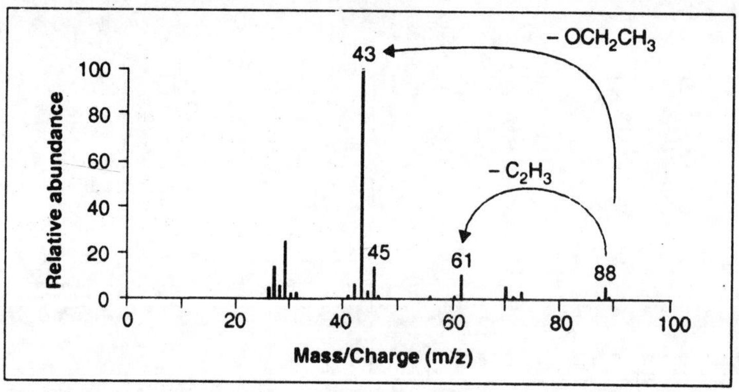

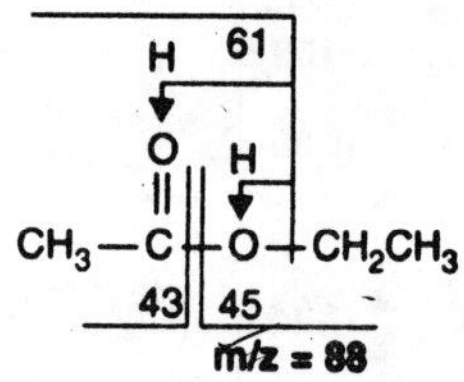

ETHER

Fragmentation tends to occur alpha to the oxygen atom (C—C bond next to the oxygen).

Ethyl methyl ether C_3H_8O **MW = 60.10**

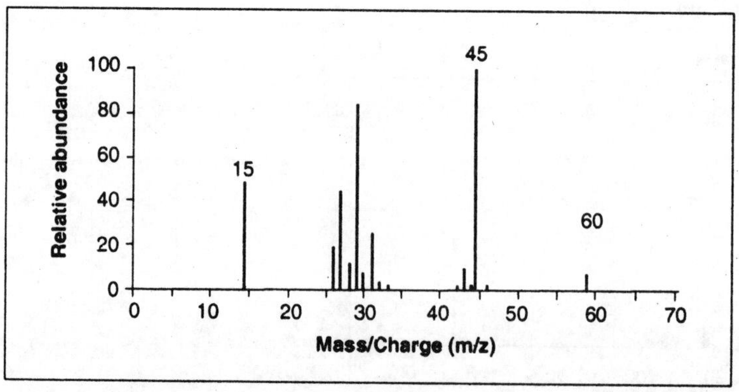

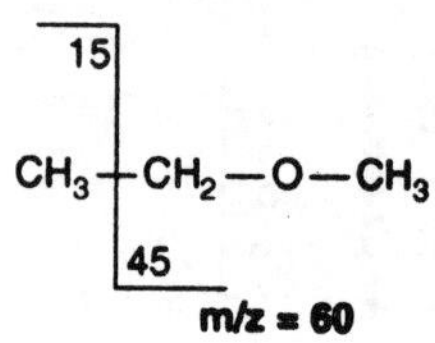

HALIDE

The presence of chlorine or bromine atoms is usually recognizable from isotopic peaks.

Bromopropane **C_3H_7Br** **MW = 123.00**

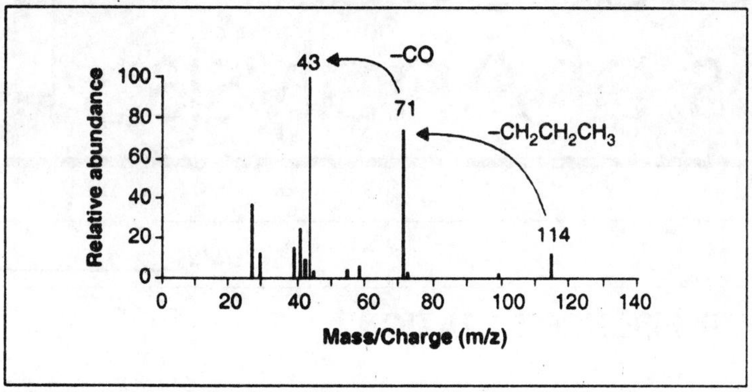

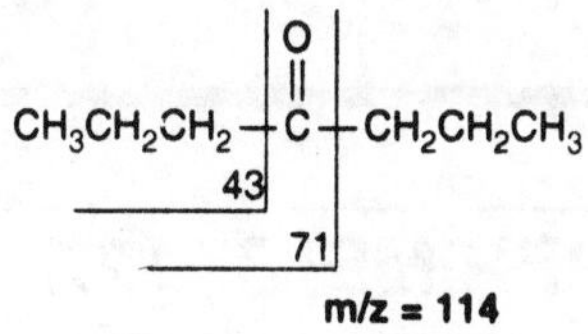

KETONE

Major fragmentation peaks result from cleavage of the C—C bonds adjacent to the carbonyl.

4-Heptanone **$C_7H_{14}O$** **MW = 114.19**

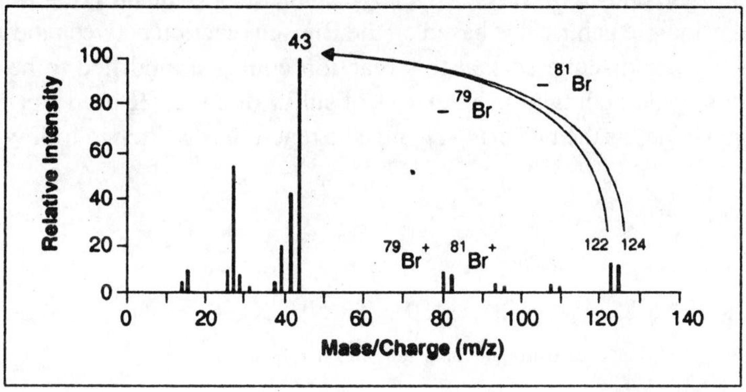

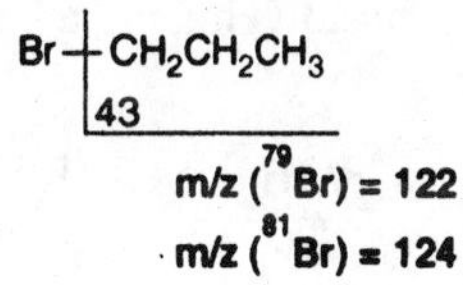

Miscellaneous Methods of Analysis

12

EXPERIMENT 12.1

Date ______________

KARL FISCHER TITRATION

AIM

To determine percentage of moisture content of the given sample by Karl Fischer titration.

PRINCIPLE

Karl Fischer titration were introduced in 1935 and are widely used analytical method for quantifying water content in a variety of products. The fundamental principle behind it is based on the Bunsen reaction between iodine and sulfur dioxide in an aqueous medium. Karl Fischer discovered that this reaction could be modified to be used for the determination of water in a non-aqueous system containing an excess of sulfur dioxide. He used a primary alcohol (methanol) as the solvent, and a base (pyridine) as the buffering agent. The reaction is written in following two parts as:

$$\underset{\text{[alcohol]}}{ROH} + SO_2\,[R'NH]SO + \underset{\text{[base]}}{R'N} \longrightarrow \underset{\text{[alkyl sulphite salt]}}{{}_3R} \quad (1)$$

$$\underset{\text{[water]}}{H_2O} + I_2\,[R'NH]SO + 2R'N + {}_3R \longrightarrow \underset{\text{[hydroiodic acid salt]}}{2[R'NH]I} + \underset{\text{[alkyl sulphate salt]}}{[R'NH]SO_4R} \quad (2)$$

In the first step alcohol reacts with sulphur dioxide (SO_2) to form ester that is neutralized by an organic base to form an intermediate alkyl sulphite salt. In the second step, which is then oxidized by iodine to an alkyl sulphate salt. This oxidation reaction consumes water. The reactive alcohol is typically methanol or 2-(2-Ethoxyethoxy)ethanol, also known as diethylene glycol monoethyl ether (DEGEE) or another suitable alcohol.

Classic Karl Fischer reagents contained pyridine (a weak base), but in currently this is replaced by imidazole or primary amines (strong base), due to the resion is that pH of the system will affect the speed and has a noxious carcinogen.

How does it work

Water and iodine are consumed in a 1:1 ratio in the above reaction. Once all of the water present is consumed, the presence of excess iodine is detected voltametrically by the titrator's indicator electrode. That signals the end-point of the titration.The amount of water present in the sample is calculated based on the concentration of iodine in the Karl Fischer titrating reagent (i.e., titer) and the amount of Karl Fischer reagent consumed in the titration.

Sensitivity of Karl Fischer Reaction against pH

The rate of the reaction depends on the pH value of the solvent, or working medium. When pH is between 5 and 8, the titration proceeds normally. However, when the pH is lower than 5, the titration speed is very slow. On the other hand, when pH is higher than 8, titration rate is fast, but only due to an interfering esterification side reaction which produces water, resulting in an vanishing endpoint. Thus, the optimal pH range for the Karl Fischer reaction is from 5 to 8, and highly acidic or basic samples need to be buffered to bring the overall pH into that range.

Types of Karl Fischer Titration

1. **Volumetric KFT**

   In volumetric Karl Fischer, iodine is added mechanically to a solvent containing the sample by the titrator's burette during the titration. Water is quantified on the basis of the volume of Karl Fischer reagent consumed. Volumetry is best suited for determination of water content in the range of 100 ppm to100%.

   There are two basic classes of volumetric KFT reagent systems:

   (*a*) **One-component volumetric KFR**, the titrating reagent (also known as a CombiTitrant, or a Composite) contains all of the chemicals needed for the Karl Fischer Reaction, namely iodine, sulphur dioxide, and the base, dissolved in a suitable alcohol. Methanol is typically used as the working medium in the titration cell. One-component volumetric reagents are easier to handle, and are usually less expensive than two-component reagents.

   (*b*) **Two-component volumetric KFR**, the titrating agent (usually known as the Titrant) contains only iodine and methanol, while the solvent containing the other Karl Fischer Reaction components is used as the working medium in the titration cell. Two-component reagents have better long-term stability and faster titration times than one-component reagents, but are usually more costly, and have lower solvent capacity.

2. **Coulometric KFT**

   In coulometric Karl Fischer, iodine is generated electrochemically *in situ* during the titration. Water is quantified on the basis of the total charge passed (Q), as measured by current (amperes) and time (seconds), according to the following relationship:

   $$Q = 1\ C\ (\text{Coulomb}) = 1\ A \times 1\ s$$

   Where $1\ mg\ H_2O = 10.72\ C$

   Coulometry is best suited for an innovative cell design is used that through a combination of factors, but without a frit, makes it nearly impossible for iodine to reach the cathode and get reduced to iodide instead of reacting with water.

How does a Volumetric Titrator work

The volumetric titrator performs the following three key functions:

1. It dispenses KF titrating reagent containing iodine into the cell using the burette.
2. It detects the endpoint of the titration using the double platinum pin indicator electrode.
3. It calculates the end result based on the volume of KF reagent dispensed using the on-board microprocessor.

How does a Coulometric Titrator work

The titrator performs the following three key functions:

1. It generates iodine at the anode of the titration cell, instead of dispensing KF reagent as in volumetric titration
2. It detects the endpoint of the titration using the double platinum pin indicator electrode.
3. It calculates the end result based on the total charge passed (Q), in coulombs, using the on-board microprocessor.

Monitoring of Titrator Performance

The use of specially formulated traceable water standards, enables efficient monitoring of titrator performance. Additionally, in volumetry, and when performing Karl Fischer titrations using an oven or evaporator, solid standards may also be used.

Standard	Form	Application(s)
Water Standard 0.01%	Liquid	Coulometry
Water Standard 0.1%	Liquid	Coulometry, Volumetry
Water Standard 1.0%	Liquid	Coulometry, Volumetry
Water Standard 5 mg/ml	Liquid	Volumetry
Water Standard Oven 1%	Solid	KF Ovens
Lactose Standard 5%	Solid	Coulometry, Volumetry, KF Ovens
Sodium Tartrate Dihydrate 15.66%	Solid	Volumetry

Selection of Sample Size

The amount of sample used depends on the anticipated water content and the desired degree of accuracy. Please refer to the following convenient reference table:

Sample Water	Volumetric	Coulometric
100%	0.02s to 0.05 g	Not recommended
50%	0.05 to 0.25 g	0.01 g
10% (1000,000 ppm)	0.25 to 0.50 g	0.01 to 0.05 g
5% (50,000 ppm)	0.50 to 2.50 g	0.05 to 0.10 g
1% (10,000 ppm)	2.50 to 5.00 g	0.10 to 0.50 g
0.5% (5,000 ppm)	5.00 to 7.50 g	0.20 to 1.00 g
0.1% (1,000 ppm)	7.50 to 10.0 g	1.00 to 2.00 g
0.01% (100 ppm)	10.0 to 15.0 g	2.00 to 5.00 g
0.001% (10 ppm)	15.0 to 20.0 g	2.00 to 5.00 g
0.0001% (1 ppm)	Not recommended	10.00 g or more

APPARATUS

Various forms of Karl Fischer apparatus for use in indirect titration are available, commercially one of general apparatus consists:

(*i*) A titration vessel of about 60 ml capacity

(*ii*) K.F. electrodes

(*iii*) Moisture trap

(*iv*) Reservoir bottle (500 ml) with burette of 10 ml capacity 0.02 ml

A titration vessel of about 60 ml capacity is fitted with two KF electrodes, a nitrogen inlet tube, a stopper which accommodates the jets of the burette and a vent tube filled with a discount such as P_2O_5 or silica gel. The substance to be examined introduced through an inlet or side arm which can be closed by a ground stopper. The stirring is done magnetically or by means of a stream of dried nitrogen passed through the solution during titration.

PROCEDURES

Primary Standardization of the Reagent

Place about 25 ml of dehydrated methyl alcohol in the titration vessels, and add sufficient Karl Fischer reagent to give the characteristic end point. Add 0.2 gm of sodium tartrate dehydrate ($C_4H_4N_2O_6 \cdot 2H_2O$) (15.66% water) accurately weighed stir and titration again with the Karl Fischer reagent. Calculate the mg of water equivalent to each ml of the K.F. reagent as:

$$\text{mg of } H_2O \text{ per ml of K.F. reagent} = \frac{\text{mg of sample} \times 0.1566}{\text{ml of reagent Karl Fischer}}$$

For example, 6.00 ml of Karl Fischer reagent is consumed by 200 mg of above sodium tartrate dehydrate sample. It means 200 mg of sodium tartrate dehydrate will have 15.66 × 200/6 × 100 of moisture. Thus each ml of reagent is capable of removing 5.22 mg of moisture. This MDF value of the reagent is 5.22.

OBSERVATION TABLE

Prepare observation table for selected quantity of sample as per guideline and availability of sample (should be 0.5 g to 2 g).

S. No.	Wt. of sample (in mg)	Burette reading (in ml) of KFR		Quantity of KFR (in ml)	Mean of nearest two values (ml)
		Initial	Final		
1.					
2.					
3.					

SAMPLE ANYLYSIS

Add about 25 ml of dehydrated methyl alcohol to the titration vessel and titrate electrochemically with Karl Fischer reagent. Transfer an accurately weighed named quantity of the sample into the titration vessel. Stir for a minute and titrate again to the electrometric endpoint Karl Fischer reagent, the water of the sample in percent is calculated as:

$$\%\text{ Moisture content} = \frac{\text{K.F. (ml)} \times \text{MDF}}{\text{Wt. of the sample in mg}} \times 100$$

Where,
MDF = Moisture deterring factor of K.F.
K.F. (ml) = K.F. reagent in ml.

If liquid sample is added, then weight of sample (mg) = vol. of the sample (ml) × specific gravity of sample. Sometime it is necessary to actually find out the moisture determination factor (MDF) of K.F. reagent. (This is done by sodium tartrate dehydrated method.)

RESULT

Percentage of moisture content of the given sample is found to be __________%.

PRECAUTIONS

1. Before filling the dehydrated methyl alcohol in titration vessel and K.F. reagent in burette, it must be necessary to remove moisture from closed set assembly by use of moisture trap.
2. After completion of experiment, it is necessary to wash all assembly with acetone to maintain the working efficiency of equipment.

EXPERIMENT 12.2

Date __________

KJELDAHL'S METHOD

AIM

To determine percentage of nitrogen content of the given sample by Kjeldahl's method.

(This method is used for determination of nitrogen contents in organic compounds.)

THEORY

The basic principle behind this is based on the digestion of organic compounds in presence of conc. H_2SO_4 and potassium sulphate or copper sulphate or potassium permagnate in a long necked round bottom flask, known as Kjeldahl flask. In presence of potassium sulphate or copper sulphate, the carbon and hydrogen of the substance get oxidized to carbon dioxide and water respectively while the nitrogen is converted into ammonia which combines with excess of the acid present to form ammonium sulphate. Initial reaction mixture colour is dark, but when reaction completed turn to colourless. The heating is then stopped and the contents of the flask are distilled with an excess of NaOH solution when the following reaction takes place:

$$C_xH_yON \xrightarrow[K_2SO_4/CuSO_4/KMnO_4]{\text{Conc. } H_2SO_4} xCO_2 + yH_2O + NH_3$$

$$NH_3 \xrightarrow{\text{Conc. } H_2SO_4} (NH_4)_2SO_4$$

$$(NH_4)_2SO_4 + 2NaOH \longrightarrow Na_2SO_4 + 2H_2O + 2NH_3$$

Unused acid is then titrated with a standard alkali solution and the amount of acid consumed in the reaction becomes known, hence the quantity of ammonia liberated in the reaction can be calculated. When we found known quantity of ammonia, calculate the percentage of nitrogen in the given organic substance that can be calculated as shown in the following example:

0.224 g of an organic substance after digesting with H_2SO_4, was distilled with an excess of NaOH solution. The liberated NH_3 gas was absorbed in 30 ml of 0.1N H_2SO_4. The excess acid left after absorption required 20 ml of 0.1N NaOH solution. Calculate the percentage of nitrogen in the substance.

20 ml of 0.1N NaOH = 20 ml of 0.1N H_2SO_4

Then, volume of 0.1N H_2SO_4 used in the neutralization of NH_3 will be = 30 – 20 = 10 ml

Weight of H_2SO_4 in 1000 ml of solution = Normality × Eq.wt.

= 0.1 × 49 = 4.9 g of H_2SO_4

30 ml of 0.1N H_2SO_4 solution contains 30 × 4.9/1000 g of H_2SO_4 = 0.147 of H_2SO_4

$$\underset{34\text{ g}}{2NH_3} + \underset{98\text{ g}}{H_2SO_4} \longrightarrow (NH_4)_2SO_4$$

According to equation, 98 g of H_2SO_4 absorbs 34 g of NH_3

0.147 g of H_2SO_4 absorbs 0.176 × 34/98 g of NH_3 = 0.051 g of NH_3

Now, 34 g NH_3 contains 28 g N_2

0.051 g NH_3 contains 0.05 × 28/34 g of NH_2 = 0.042 g of N_2

Since, 0.224 g of substance contains 0.042 g N_2

100 g substance contains 100 × 0.042/0.224 g N_2 = 18.75%

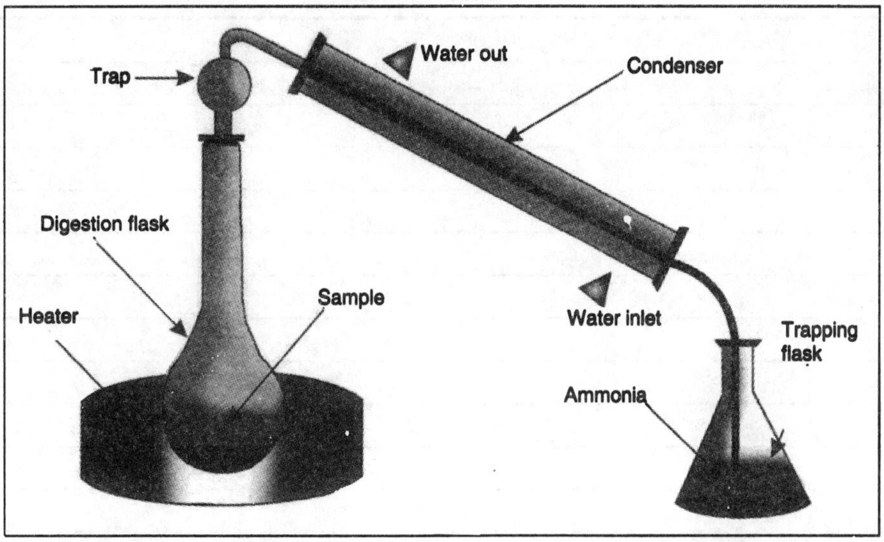

OBSERVATION TABLE

S. No.	Amount of sample taken (g)	Quantity of 0.1 N H_2SO_4 taken	0.1 N NaOH solution used (ml)		Quantity of excess 0.1 N H_2SO_4 remain in flask after titration
			Initial (ml)	Final (ml)	

NOTES

1. Reason behind addition of potassium, mercury, cadmium and copper either in combined or calculated form to increase the boiling point of the sulphuric acid and catalyze the oxidation of organic compounds.
2. Kjeldahl's method is unsatisfactory for estimation of nitrogen present azo, nitro, cyano, hydrazo and on heterocycles.
3. This is suitable for determination of nitrogen content in organic amines or amides.

Reader's Notes